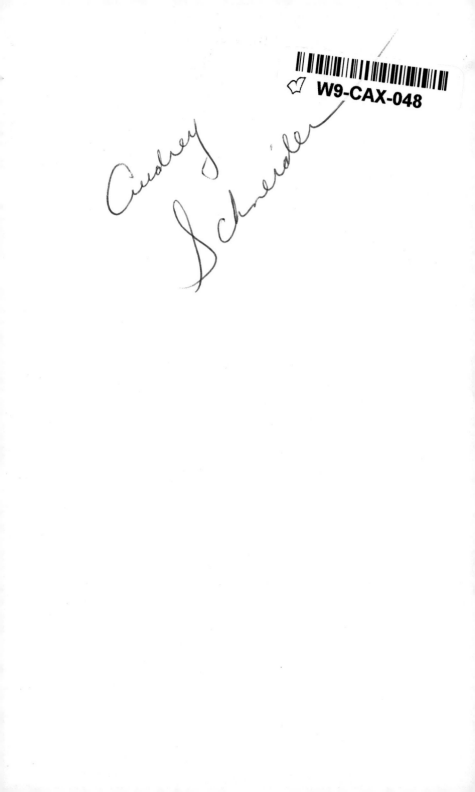

W9-CAX-048

Is It Hot in Here or Is It Me?

Is It Hot in Here
or Is It Me?

A PERSONAL LOOK AT THE FACTS, FALLACIES, AND FEELINGS OF MENOPAUSE

Gayle Sand

FOREWORD BY Morris Notelovitz, M.D., Ph.D.

HarperCollins*Publishers*

HarperCollins books may be purchased for educational, business, or sales promotional use. For information please write: Special Markets Department, HarperCollins Publishers, Inc., 10 East 53rd Street, New York, NY 10022.

A STONEWORK

FIRST EDITION

Designed by Barbara Du Pree Knowles

LIBRARY OF CONGRESS CATALOGING-IN-PUBLICATION DATA

Sand, Gayle.
    Is it hot in here or is it me? : a personal look at the facts, fallacies, and feelings of menopause / Gayle Sand; foreword by Morris Notelovitz.—1st ed.
        p.   cm.
    Includes index.
    ISBN 0-06-018341-1
    1. Menopause—Popular works.   I. Title.
    RG186.S26   1993   92-54734
    612.6′65—dc20

93 94 95 96 97 CC/HC 10 9 8 7 6 5 4 3 2 1

Contents

CONTENTS

Acknowledgments

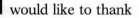 would like to thank

My editor, HarperCollins Vice President and Associate Publisher Gladys Justin Carr, for her belief in me and her unbelievable editorial skills, and Editorial Associate Tracy Devine, who truly is—for always being there for me and helping make some tough choices.

Jeff Stone and Jane Friedman for all their help in getting me started.

Dr. Morris Notelovitz for thoroughly examining my manuscript and giving it a clean bill of health.

All those patient doctors and health care professionals who answered my never-ending stream of questions—Theresa Galsworthy, Dr. Phyllis Adler, Tina Dieno, Dr. Shirley Hartman, Win Smith, Marcus Laux, N.D., Dr. John Lee, and especially the knowledgeable and caring Dr. Michael Sanders, my menopause sparring partner.

ACKNOWLEDGMENTS

All the women who shared their menopause with me—your names have been changed but you know who you are. Diane English, up front with her own name.

Rod "Jez" Leonard, who started the computer work, and Lee Cisar, who finished it and finished it and finished it until it became the start of a great friendship.

My friends who cut, clipped, faxed, pasted, copied, taped, recorded, encouraged, and sent me information—my sister, Meryl Lavine, Jean Gordon, Lynda Sheldon, Andy Port, Patrick Higgins, Cindy Spoerle, Kathleen Steed, Nancy Rica Schiff, Laura Skoler, Diane Thomas, Bob Sleight, George Klabin, Harold George, Steve Stangle, Janice Brown, Crystal Bretz, Candy Konrath, Tracey Deputy, Christa Hofer, Miles Ingram, Tom Wiley, Karen Lynch, Kevin Schmidt, Suzie Tannous, Len Lapsys, Paul Rubinstein, Jack Uram, Bunny Hart, Joann Speranza, Wayne Mundy, and Jane Meisel.

Dr. Jack Chachkes, my best friend and chief cheerleader whose daily dose of encouragement was like a shot in the arm.

Hayden, for your quiet support and affection.

And especially my husband—for his love, sense of humor, and for not allowing my change of life to change our life.

Foreword

Why is it that after all this time a natural part of a woman's life, the menopause, has become the subject of magazine articles and landed on bestseller lists? Why is a normal and inescapable part of being a woman now a media subject and, equally important, in danger of becoming "medicalized"? By describing her own personal experience, Gayle Sand has performed a valuable service, offering an uninhibited, real look at what is a universal journey for women and their companions.

Is It Hot in Here or Is It Me? gives readers a unique perspective on a subject that daily is getting more attention; yet few even understand the term "menopause." Menopause itself refers to a woman's last menstrual period, a passage of no more than a week. The hormonal and other subtle changes referred to as "the change of life" do not happen in the final week of menstruation but precede and postdate this time by nearly fifteen years in either direction. This entire passage of about thirty years is known as "the climacteric" and, like puberty—another period of great physiological change—it results in certain physical changes and symptoms. It is *this* that all the concern is about.

The climacteric has become the focus of talk shows and other public forums for two important reasons: First, 42 million women in this year alone will be experiencing the climacteric; second, the baby boomers are growing up. This is a generation that has always questioned things and often discovered that initial answers were suspect and frequently wrong. They are not content with the same advice their mothers were given. The emotional roller coaster and at times physical discomfort that often manifest themselves during the climacteric were not, for this generation, going to be dealt with by a simple "this is natural, the way it's always been" attitude—in other words, grin and bear it. This new generation of women recognizes that each woman experiences her own menopause, just like the individual experience of childbirth, or marriage, or work. As these previous points in life vary from one woman to another, so too are the differences each woman feels in going through menopause.

No matter how different the experience is for every woman, however, two basic questions still remain: "How are you doing?" and "Do you need help?" This book attempts to answer both of those questions. Gayle with her at-the-kitchen-table-with-a-cup-of-coffee style shares her journey with both humor and insight. Her journey provides the reader with a well-researched investigation of the menopause. Gayle asked and received answers to many questions involving her menopause. She went to a broad spectrum of health care providers, from Madison Avenue gynecologists to New Age healers. She tried out their recommendations, experienced the response, and came to her own conclusions.

Gayle's initial instinct was correct: Menopause is an inevitable milestone in life and though sometimes difficult, it is not a disease. Consequently, her suspicion of the physician and of the potential medicalization of menopause was understandable. She knew good health depended on knowledge as well as on taking care of oneself. Checkups are a sensible precaution that allow a woman to make better decisions and to be involved with her own preventative health care.

Gayle, in her transition into menopause, made a number of important personal discoveries. She didn't come to them alone, but shared and experienced them with her husband. Gayle's wisdom was not only in questioning and obtaining medical advice, but equally important in involving her husband. I can attest to the latter, not only as a physician but as a postmenopausal husband myself. The message to be gotten from Gayle's experience is to involve the rest of your crew—husband, children, significant other, friends, and associates. They will help a singular experience become plural.

This book is funny. It is written with a sense of humor about something people aren't used to laughing about. Beyond the humor, the pleasure of reading *Is It Hot in Here or Is It Me?* lies in its serious truths based on good research. Gayle writes about real facts defined by our present understanding and her own personal experience. Hormone therapy is not necessary for everyone, but in many instances it can be a veritable lifesaver.

Gayle's book helps turn the questions and uncertainties of menopause into a wonderful story that all of us can relate to and enjoy. No one ever claimed menopause was a laughing matter, but Gayle comes pretty close; and even the medical community recognizes that laughter can be the best medicine of all.

Morris Notelovitz, M.D., Ph.D.

Morris Notelovitz is an internationally recognized authority in the field of gynecology and climacteric medicine. He is the founder and president of the Women's Medical and Diagnostic Center in Gainesville, Florida, and founded the nation's first center for the study of the climacteric (menopause) at the University of Florida in 1976. In addition to serving on numerous medical and editorial boards and societies, Dr. Notelovitz is a member of the U.S. congressional advisory panels on menopause, hormone replacement therapy, and osteoporosis.

Introduction

When you think of Raquel Welch, Diana Ross, Sophia Loren, and Jane Fonda, do you also think of vaginal dryness, hot flashes, night sweats, heart disease, and the bone-thinning disease osteoporosis? Well, I do. Because it makes me feel better knowing that these famous, sexy, successful women are going through what I'm going through, menopause.

Menopause, the end of one's menstrual cycle, is an equal-opportunity employer. It happens to all women. It's a sure thing like death and taxes. There is nothing exclusive or exotic about it. This isn't a ride on the space shuttle or a cruise to Tahiti. This is a trip every woman gets to experience. For some it will be smooth sailing, for others it will be as scary as a jump on a bungee cord. Whether you live in Beverly Hills or Belgrade, Manhattan or Marrakesh, sooner or later you'll be riding the Menopause Express.

All your life you might have been out of touch with your body but at menopause you'll start hearing from it. Things will start to happen. Your periods will stop. You might get hair on your face. Sex can become painful and you may even lose your desire for desire. Hot flashes? A definite possibility. Night sweats and insomnia? Often. Urinary tract infections? Not uncommon. Depression and mood swings? Could happen. Fortunately, for most women the prognosis isn't psychosis.

Menopause can even be a relief. No more periods can mean no more worries about menstrual cramps, bloating, bleeding problems, the price of tampons or birth control. It can also be a freeing, liberating experience. For some reason everyone expects you to go a little looney at menopause. So now you can say and do pretty much anything you want and all you have to do is blame it on menopause. When your in-laws come to visit, stay in bed watching TV the whole time they're there. When they ask what's wrong, blame it on menopause. They'll understand. Gain five pounds? Blame it on menopause and you'll get sympathetic nods. Bounce a check, send back the main course, return a tasteless gift, disagree with your mother, leave the house without makeup. No problem. All you have to do is blame it on menopause. It's expected. You're allowed to go off your rocker and lose it. The only problem is, no woman in her right mind wants the whole world knowing she's getting old. It's bad for her image.

Thanks to Madison Avenue and the medical community, the image of the menopausal woman was a ma-
tronly, sexless female whose shopping list included Poli-
dent, Metamucil, Geritol, and Attends. The menopausal
woman was a red-faced, white-gloved, blue-haired, all-
American joke, whose hair got caught in an Eisenhower
time warp and whose Lycra tights had melted into Supp-
Hose. I'm not that Madison Avenue woman and neither
are my friends.

I was scared to death of becoming a menopausal
woman. Losing my period was traumatic. It was a change
I couldn't accept, so I denied it. I wasn't losing my period,
it was just late. Not over, just on sabbatical. I continued
using birth control and buying Tampax when it was on
sale. They were my reproductive ID cards and I couldn't
accept the fact that they were no longer valid. I never
talked to anyone about it. The longer I didn't talk about
it the more isolated I became. The more isolated I became
the crazier I got. I started making deals with God. "Give
me back my period and I'll call my parents every week."
God wasn't making any deals. I was menopausal and I
realized it was time to accept my menopause and deal
with it.

Although I have always tried to experience rather
than read about life, in this case I ran to books to find out
anything I could. I found out about the symptoms but
little about the human aspect of this time in my life. Every
book I looked at had the emotion and humor of the latest

issue of *Popular Mechanics*. There was plenty of information, but very little commiseration. It was going to take more than maxims to master menopause. There was no simple step-by-step solution. This was going to take trial and a lot of error.

My menopausal journey lasted three years, and was experienced in L.A., New York, and St. Augustine, Florida. During that time I consulted everyone who knew anything about menopause—hormonal agnostics, estrogen zealots, Christian Scientists, Seventh-Day Adventists, recovering hippies, hypochondriacs, Rosicrucians—you name it. I talked to elders, crones, wisewomen, midwives, gynecologists, and gurus to get the lowdown on estrogen slowdown. I tried everything from acupuncture to Zen Buddhism. I was a patient patient, got hundreds of "second" opinions, and was referred to enough doctors to suffer refer madness. I've been to healers who tried to relieve my vaginal dryness with crystals, prayer, and the laying on of hands, a nutritionist who determined my calcium levels by reading my pubic hair, and an ayurvedic doctor who made the frequency of my hot flashes go from four a day to thirty a day. I've been measured, tested, bled, scanned, rayed, wired, picked, poked, advised, and prescribed. I have seen more gynecologists and climbed into more stirrups than Dale Evans and Roy Rogers combined. I have tried to learn everything about the flashes, the flushes, the minuses, the pluses, the facts, the fads, the pros, the cons, the ins, the outs, the ups, the downs, the emotion, and the commotion of menopause.

I was new at this. I wasn't aware of the options and I made many mistakes. I ad-libbed my way through it but you don't have to. When I experienced my first hot flash, menopause was a world of quiet denial. Women didn't talk about menopause. It was a deep dark secret lost in the Bermuda Triangle of women's problems. What silicone did for implants, Watergate for Nixon, cholesterol for meat, Anita Hill for Clarence Thomas, menopause did for middle age. It gave it a bad name. Women were reluctant to share the experience. Thankfully, my friends broke the silence and helped me through the confusion and fear. What I hope to accomplish with this book is to share my experiences with you and be there for you the way they were for me. Menopause is a journey best shared and thankfully more of us are now sharing.

And just as we're quick to teach younger generations the facts of life, we must also fill them in on the facts of change of life. I certainly would have been much better equipped to handle it if I had known earlier on what I know now. Exercise and diet and other life-style changes can have a major effect on your menopause, and the sooner you make them the better. The ideal time to learn about menopause is not when you are going through it, but when you are in your twenties and thirties and can do the most about it.

In the three years since my first hot flash I have gone through some profound personal changes, but they are nothing compared to the changes going on around me. When I first got a hot flash nobody talked about menopause. Now everybody is talking. Menopause is the hot new topic. The hot flash has replaced the cold war. Menopause is on more lips than oat bran, and estrogen therapy is the new co-dependency. Now it is in to be out of estrogen. Menopause has come out of the dark recesses of middle age and into the bright light of daytime TV. Everywhere you look old wives are telling their tales about menopause. Everybody is now naming names, saying sayings, and revealing revelations. Menopause has arrived. Midlife has met the mainstream. Hormones have hit the heartland.

Now there are newsletters, hotlines, seminars, workshops, and support groups. Menopause is the subject of best-selling books, features in scented upscale magazines, and articles in big-city and small-town newspapers. I just saw a full-page ad for the Estraderm patch—not in *Modern Maturity*, but in *U.S.A. Today*. We are in the middle of a change-of-life movement and with good reason. In the next two decades, more than 40 million American women will be experiencing menopause. The baby boom generation is rapidly approaching the "Big M." It is hard to keep 40 million boomers silent.

It won't be long before there will be a Beverly Hills

Polo and Menopause Club, Night Sweat Cruises to
Alaska, menopause boutiques, and a hot new fragrance
from some menopausal movie star called "Flash." Yes,
the times they are changing. As my megatrend manicurist, Ramona, says, "Nobody is doing youth these days."
Menopause is hot, it's hip, it's it, it's in, it's happening,
it's now. For the nineties, it's menopause, uh-*huh!* Go
figure.

Is It Hot in Here or Is It Me?

First Flash

I experienced my first hot flash in Los Angeles at a very trendy sports club where they have a machine for everything except menopause. If you thought your body was a temple then Sports Club L.A. is Mecca with valet parking. It's a square block of postmodern glass and steel devoted to the worship of perfect fitness, the adoration of spandex, and the elimination of cellulite.

When I first stepped inside the place I couldn't believe it. It was health heaven. Saunas, Jacuzzis, steam rooms, swimming pool, track, health bar, tanning salon, boutique, and rows and rows of color coordinated exercise machines designed to work every body part from your little pinky to your big toe. Everything was bigger and better than anything I had ever seen before. This was no ordinary gym. This was a gym on steroids.

Upstairs in the aerobic section rich guys in Reeboks

and Rolexes rowed like galley slaves, while captains of industry made deals on their cellular phones as they climbed the StairMaster. There were celebrities everywhere. Some were easy to spot. Dyan Cannon wore a weight belt that spelled her name in four-inch block letters, just in case you didn't know who she was. Others were more difficult to identify. A constant chant echoed through the gym. "Who's that? Who's that? Who's that?"

It was all very intimidating, but most intimidating was the locker room. You are naked and you are surrounded by very young, very tanned women, breasts at attention, buns bearing magnetic north, posing for some imaginary camera. This was no place for amateurs. Here you had to be in shape just to get in shape. At my previous "club," the Twenty-third Street YMCA in New York, I was considered a 10. Here I am lucky if I'm a 5. The women wear full makeup, designer spandex, and they never sweat. I took an aerobics class with them five times a week.

On this day the aerobics class had a new instructor. Not more than ten minutes into the class I started to sweat profusely. As rivulets of my sweat started forming dark blue puddles on the light blue carpet I thought, Boy, this instructor is great. When I looked around it was obvious that nobody else was sharing my experience. The pink spandex to my right was bone-dry and her carpet was still light blue. The gold Rolex to my left didn't have a bead of perspiration on her face. When I realized I was all alone my heart started doing a flamenco dance against my chest. It felt like my thermostat had been kicked. Perrier was pouring out of me. The more attention I paid to the sweating the hotter I got. I felt like I was in the sauna. I kept looking at the smoke alarm above me praying I wouldn't set it off. What could it be? Faulty sweat glands? Malaria? Could this be global warming? I hoped so. Then as quickly as it came it went away.

Later that day I was shopping at Gelson's supermarket. As I opened the glass and metal door of the frozen food locker I was hit with a blast of fake Arctic air and once again I felt that warm clammy feeling and my heart started dancing. Here I am leaning into a freezer, surrounded by rock-hard boxes of frozen foods, and I am defrosting! I had been in this case a thousand times and nothing like this had ever happened. Obviously it wasn't that new aerobics instructor. What could it be? Could I be having a hot flash? Aren't hot flashes and heart palpitations one of the first signs of menopause? I remember reading Gail Sheehy's book *Passages,* in which she described the waves of heat and chills. They are called vasomotor instability and they occur when the brain's temperature-regulating center goes haywire, causing blood vessels that are near the skin to dilate, which triggers a rush of heat and perspiration. But is this possible? I'm only forty-seven years old and a member of Sports Club L.A. Maybe it is. Maybe that missed period wasn't too much exercise. Maybe this experience is a hot flash. Maybe I'm beginning menopause. I panicked. In L.A. nobody experiences menopause. In L.A. menopause is considered a terminal illness.

As I wheel my cart to the checkout counter I pass rows of neatly stacked, perfectly ripe apples and plums and peaches and pears. The produce at Gelson's is selected very carefully. It is then washed and buffed and shined until it is moist and wet and beautiful. If it is overripe or blemished, or flawed even in the slightest way, it is thrown out.

In L.A. women are treated a lot like produce and their shelf life is about the same as a quart of milk. Here they appreciate vintage wine, respect old money, collect antique cars, and trade in menopausal women. L.A. is definitely not a menopause town. If it were, women would be driving around with vanity license plates that read HT FLSH R or CHGE O LIFR or O.PERIOD. In L.A. you "do" lunch, not menopause.

When I walk outside Gelson's it is cool and dry. I am hot and wet. I now have my own weather. I haven't sweated this much since the time I missed my period and thought I was pregnant. I keep asking, "What is this? What is going on? What is happening?" It is the first time

I have talked to myself in many years. Until now I had no reason to. Since puberty, everything had been going just fine.

I am upset and puzzled by the Gelson's experience. When I get in my car I calmly roll up the windows, scream at the top of my lungs, fasten my seat belt, and drive home. Home for me and my husband is one of the many luxury high-rise apartment buildings that form a corridor along Wilshire Boulevard. In this part of L.A. even the buildings are in show business. They compete for attention by offering glamorous amenities like uniformed doormen and valet parking and concierge and health clubs. All have breathtaking views of the traffic. On smog-alert days the view is even more breathtaking.

Our building has one hundred apartments and parking for five hundred. I pull into the cavernous, immaculately clean, air-conditioned indoor garage. I am still troubled by the day's events. I decide to work off my anxieties. I put away the groceries, change into my sweats, and make my way to our building's health club. The "club" is a small, windowless room directly behind the flashy lobby. It is equipped with an obsolete training bike, a slant board, a $1.98 bogus Universal machine, a Ping-Pong table, and a Jacuzzi that hasn't worked since we moved in a year ago. A faded sign on the Jacuzzi reads

"Pardon the Inconvenience." As usual the club is empty. Most of the tenants prefer walking their cars. I get on the bike. I start pedaling and thinking about what just happened to me and my body.

Lillian Hellman said, "People change and they forget to tell each other." Well, sometimes people change and they forget to tell themselves. Take me and my body for example. We go back forty-seven years and from the very beginning we were in touch. We communicated. We were there for each other. When we were just a few weeks old if my body was wet or hungry it told me and we cried. If it was bloated we burped. When I was nine months old and wanted to get from point A to point B vertically, like a team we worked on the problem together and in no time we advanced from crawling to walking. The arrangement worked just fine and together we got through measles, mumps, puberty, and adolescence.

We built on our relationship. The longer we were together the better we communicated. We were linked, coupled, connected. It took care of me and I took care of it. Sure, we had our disagreements. Certain foods got it very upset and certain people made it nauseated. But we adjusted. We stopped eating anchovies and lamb chops and cough drops and pickled herring. I was a good provider. I bought my body nothing but the best foods, lotions, and shampoos. I never abused it. When it was tired we rested. I sacrificed for it. I worked overtime to pay for tennis lessons and mambo lessons and massages. But my body was worth it.

I know I wasn't perfect. That New Year's Eve when I ate the whole cherry cheesecake and the weekend in Atlantic City with that half gallon of Häagen-Dazs Rum Raisin. But we made up for it. Those evenings when I would come home late from work, dead tired, and we'd go out and jog. Or those freezing cold winter mornings when we'd get up at 5:00 A.M. to go to the gym. Sure it was tough, but we needed exercise. I wasn't crazy about jogging but we did what was good for my body.

In the '60s we followed Adelle Davis. And we were what we ate. We read Dr. Walker and we juiced our way to health. I even bought an expensive juicer just so we would have sixty-four ounces of fresh juice every day. We were in it together. In the '70s it was vitamin C with Linus Pauling and Dr. Frank's No Aging Diet. Who else but us would stick five cans of skinless and boneless, packed-in-water, no-salt-added sardines down our throat every week. Sardines make me gag, but that was okay. A small price to pay for our great skin and great memory. I really cared for my body. Sometimes, I went to extreme lengths to keep it healthy. I'd bring my own food to greasy-spoon restaurants. Sure, I made enemies at the restaurant and I insulted and embarrassed my dinner companions. But that was okay. I was willing to take the heat because we were partners. We were a team like Thelma and Louise,

George and Gracie, and Cagney and Lacey. We went together like a car and driver, a horse and rider.

Our relationship was more than just physical. We were in sync. We were in touch. And then out of nowhere, without as much as a whimper or a warning, I am having hot flashes. The nerve of my body to change and not clear it with me first!

I stop pedaling and get off the bike. I have worked out but I am still worked up. My body took me for a ride and now I'm going to take it for a walk to Westwood Village to get even. There's a Taco Bell there and I'm going to drown my sorrows in heavy doses of burritos, fries, and chocolate chip cookies. Then I am going to 7–Eleven and wash it all down with a Slurpy. We're talking, at a minimum, 3,500 calories' worth of abuse. I walk through the overchandeliered, glass-walled, popcorn-plastered lobby and out onto Wilshire Boulevard.

I am dwarfed by my surroundings. In L.A. when you are not driving everything appears overscaled. The street is too wide, the blocks too long, the sidewalks too narrow. It is designed for tires, not shoes. The perspective is off. It is all too big. I feel very small. As I walk the gauntlet of new high-rises, I am aware of the long, striped, brightly colored canopies stretching from their doorways. I get the feeling that the buildings are sticking their tongues out at me. They should treat me with more respect. I am older than all of them.

When I finally get to Westwood Village I can't go through with it. I wind up at Penguin's Yogurt, sample the peanut butter crunch, and settle for a small cup of nonfat, sugar-free French vanilla. It is twelve calories an ounce. It tastes like 3,500. Nonfat frozen yogurt, the miracle of the '80s.

A lot of New Yorkers think that yogurt is the only culture in L.A. This is only partially correct. There is also the mall bookstore and its cousin, the multiplex theater. The Beverly Center has all three. I guess you could call it L.A.'s answer to New York's Lincoln Center. I drive there to buy a book about menopause. I need more information. Maybe I'm overreacting, maybe I'm jumping to conclusions.

The book store is near the multiplex theater. When I enter it is crowded with moviegoers killing time until the next show. An Armani-clad agent type stands by the magazine rack making dinner reservations on his cellular phone, while his Armani-clad thirteen-year-old heavily-moussed son studies the pictures of the naked cars in the *Robb Report*. I weave past a middle-aged man reading a middle-aged book by John Updike as I work my way to the health section.

The shelves are stuffed with copies of *The 8-Week Cholesterol Cure*. It is written by Robert E. Kowalski. He is only forty-one and he has already had a heart attack and two bypass operations. I think to myself: "I wept because I had no period until I met a woman who had no uterus." It doesn't work. This fails to put things in perspective. I want an eight-week menopause cure.

I pick up a biography of Angela Lansbury. I immediately turn to the index and look under "Lansbury, Angela Brigid . . . marriage of . . . motherhood of . . ." There is no "menopause of." I flip through a copy of *Elizabeth Takes Off*. In it Liz Taylor talks openly and honestly about everything except menopause. I see a book called *Misery*, by Stephen King. The title sounds like it could be about menopause. But the author tells me I'm dreaming. Surely, there must be a book about menopause, even in L.A.

I walk boldly to the counter and at the bottom of my lungs I whisper, "Do you have anything on menopause?" The clerk, a young girl with perfect features, leans toward me.

"Metaphors?" she asks with the innocence of youth. I am tempted to say yes, metaphors, but I don't.

"Menopause," I say a little louder.

"Menopause," she repeats a little louder. "Let me check." I wince as she punches the keys on her computer. I now have emotional recall. I feel like I'm fifteen and in the grocery story buying my first Kotex. "I show nothing," the clerk says. A few people waiting to pay for their books line up behind me. They are now in earshot.

I stare at Hillary's name tag as she turns to her supervisor. "Jeffrey, help me with this. Do we have anything on menopause for this woman?"

Mortified, I stare straight ahead as Jeffrey jabs the keys of his terminal, repeating "Menopause . . . menopause . . . menopause . . ." as he scans the screen. I want this torture to end. I want Jeffrey to go to his neutral corner and leave me alone. Just as I am about to throw in the towel Jeffrey looks up and smiles. "We have a book called *Menopause: A Positive Approach,* by Rosetta Reitz."

I avoid all eye contact as he leads me past the staring crowd to the paperback section. When I pay for the book I jokingly ask him to put it in a brown paper bag. Nobody laughs. As I leave, Hillary asks me if I want my parking ticket validated. "Yes, thank you," I say gratefully. Validation is something I really need right now.

So when out of the blue I get a call from my old friend, Stanley, I am very receptive. I have not seen Stanley in twenty-five years. We grew up in the same middle-class neighborhood in Queens. He was big and dark and tough and cute. All the girls thought he looked like Tony Curtis. When he married Gina and I married Jerome, my first husband, we lost touch. He heard I was now living in Los Angeles and would like to take me to dinner and talk about old times. I have always liked Stanley and I am curious to see what became of him. "Sure," I say. As I hang up the phone the word "old" keeps ringing in my ears.

We meet at a Japanese restaurant on the second floor of a shopping center in Westwood. It is one of those places that has vivid color pictures of the sushi on the walls. It's about as appetizing as the Most Wanted mug-shots in the post office. Stanley has lost a little hair and gained a lot of weight. He is about sixty pounds heavier than when I last saw him. He is still big and dark and tough and cute, but now he looks less like Tony Curtis and more like Paul Sorvino. The old Stanley wore blue jeans and Aqua-Velva. Today's Stanley is dressed all in black and wears Giorgio for Men. The restaurant staff greets him warmly. They know him well. It is obvious that this place has made a major contribution to Stanley's increased circumference. As we are led to a table I make sure that we are seated at one close to an air-conditioning duct. I am taking no chances.

Once seated we nervously play with our chopsticks as we tell each other the required how-great-we-look and how-little-we've-changed. Then Stanley leans across the table and gets down to some serious business. He tells me about this incredible crush he used to have on me. I am surprised, flattered, and uncomfortable. "How come you never let me know?" I ask.

"You know how uptight we were back in the '50s.

If a guy liked a girl he'd have a party, invite everybody, including her, and then talk to everybody at the party but her. We were so indirect then, so stupid, so dishonest, so . . ." I am sitting opposite a middle-aged man relating to me like a teenage boy. Stanley is suffering from suspended adoration. His feelings are frozen in time. That's what happens when you haven't seen someone in twenty-five years. The same thing happened at my high school reunion. Jerks were still considered jerks even if they were major success stories. They might be brain surgeons to the outside world, but to us they were still Mr. Whoopee Cushion. I am tempted to tell him that this "girl" he had a crush on is experiencing menopause. I don't. I'm enjoying the time warp.

The waiter arrives. Stanley orders in Japanese. He speaks fluent menu. I change the subject. "How's Gina?" He tells me that he's getting a divorce, that she is ripping him off, that business is lousy, that he's dangerously over-weight, and he couldn't be happier. Obviously he is a man experiencing midlife crisis. To relieve the sexual tension, I tell him about my new husband and my happy new marriage, emphasizing the word happy. I make no mention of my happy new hot flashes. The food arrives. It is sushi for forty. Stanley is not at all intimidated.

I ask him if he's seeing anybody. "Everybody," he says. He then goes on to tell me about his new liberated sex life that includes whips and chains and bondage and pain on the bed, under the bed, and tied to the bed. Stanley is a regular buccaneer. I am eating sushi with Captain Horatio Hornblower. As the Captain tells me of his exploits I nod my head like I've been there. In truth, what I have done in this area is the equivalent of a hickey. Men and women approach midlife differently. I feel I am losing my libido and his is out of control.

Uneasy with the direction our conversation is taking, I make a segue from Mars. "Do you think chlorophyll was the oat bran of the '50s?" No response. He devours an entire California roll. I press on. "Remember chloro-phyll dog food?" Nothing. "Remember the great challah French toast at the La Salle Diner on Queens Boulevard?" He stops chewing.

"How about the blueberry knishes on the board-walk at Long Beach?" he adds playfully. We are both a lot more comfortable in this area of high-calorie nos-talgia. Now names and places bounce between us with the pop and clang and clatter of an old pinball machine. Friends that dropped out, others that sold out, soap on a rope and losers on dope, cardiac arrest and est, passion pits and face lifts, excess, success, and tilt. We are ex-hausted and so is the food supply. Stanley pays the check in fluent American Express and we leave.

Outside, the parking attendant gets Stanley's car. It is a beige Mercedes convertible. Stanley reaches in and hands me a videotape. "Watch this, you'll get a big kick out of it," he says. I take the tape and give him a big hug. As he gets in his car he poses behind the wheel. "Hey, is this me or what?"

"Stanley, you're not short, sleek, beige, and German," I say as he drives off.

When I get home my husband is asleep. I decide to preview the tape because I'm thinking it's probably a home movie of Stanley the Buccaneer, a German shepherd, and a French maid. Stanley's sex life is wild enough to be X-rated and mine is tame enough to be on America's Funniest Home Videos. I put the tape in the machine and hope for the best.

It is a grainy, 8mm home movie that has been transferred to videotape. It is of Stanley and Gina and me and Jerome on Long Beach in the summer of 1963. We are all thin and tan and goofy. I am sporting an Aqua-Net-stiff foot-high beehive and Cleopatra eyeliner. Stanley, in Dippity-Dooed hair, removes a cigarette from behind his ear and lights up as Gina barbecues herself with a reflector and Jerome bastes in a sauce of iodine and baby oil. We self-consciously make faces at the camera with our behinds as it searches frantically to put something, anything on film.

I am watching me at twenty-two and for some reason I am not affected in the way I thought I would be. I don't cry. I don't get emotional. But I do examine carefully and critically the girl in the beehive and the kelly-green bikini. Except for the loss of a couple of pounds of hair and eyeliner, it doesn't appear that I have changed that much. In fact, I think I look better now.

Immediately after viewing the tape, while the image is still fresh in my mind, I walk to the mirror and look carefully at myself. I am very pleased with what I see. Mirror, mirror on the wall: "Is this me or what?" Or am I short, sleek, beige, and German also?

Healing and Dealing

When I was fourteen years old, I was insecure. My friends had breasts. I didn't. They were in bras; I was in Fruit of the Loom. They were getting their periods; I was getting impatient. I was so insecure that I even pretended. I would ask for a nickel for the Kotex machine, pop a couple of ersatz Midol, complain of cramps, and go home.

It is thirty-three years later. And my little menstrual show continues. I am a mature, worldly woman of forty-seven and I am doing basically the same thing. I no longer get my periods and again I'm insecure about it. I don't pop fake Midol but I do buy real Tampax whenever it's on sale. I even keep a supply in my locker at the gym. If anybody needs a Tampax I'm the first to offer. I hand them out like they're cocktail franks. "Here, have a Tampax."

I couldn't continue with this denial and deception. I had to face up to the fact that I was missing my periods. I was having hot flashes and heart palpitations and my night sweats were keeping me up half the night. I was irritable and cranky. And to top it off, the inside of my vagina had suddenly developed a sandpaper texture like a cat's tongue, making sex very painful. A perfect environment for my husband's penis if he were the Marquis de Sade. To stop the dryness I used so much K-Y Jelly that my vagina had the consistency of a strawberry shortcake. The ecstasy just wasn't worth the agony or the mess. The high levels of pain led to low levels of lust.

One morning after a particularly bad, sleepless, uncomfortable night of meltdowns and turn-downs, I turn on the TV. I watch as an immaculately groomed, beautiful, shapely, gray-haired woman talks about her menopause experience. She begins with the old Norman Vincent Peale stuff. "I didn't get older. I got better." And then she goes on to extol the wonders of menopause. The freedom, the zest, the unlimited sexual and social and spiritual opportunities available to the menopausal woman. The audience, consisting of young women and unemployed men, applaud after every one of her outrageous statements while the host tells the guest how wonderful she is and how great she looks. Based on what I have just seen you would think that menopause is a resort in the Bahamas and that the experience is pretty much a sun-baked, fun-filled cruise. I turn off the TV.

I sit there exhausted with a pounding headache, damp and cranky from an evening of night sweats, a dry aching vagina, and a crushed libido. I think to myself, Do I live on the same planet as this woman I have just seen on TV? Or is there something wrong with me? Am I really suffering? Or am I just neurotic and imagining things? Are there any other earthlings out there like me?

It was time to see a doctor. Dr. Matz is our family physician. He is an internist with an office in one of those L.A. professional medical buildings, filled with well-heeled patients who aren't healing well. Plenty of doctors. Plenty of parking. Cars drive in and old people shuffle out. A lot of young nurses in white helping old people in pain fill out Medicare forms. For the first time in my life I can identify with the shuffling, C-shaped patients. We are all in the same boat. They have just been in it a lot longer.

Dr. Matz gives me a very thorough examination and I tell him everything that is going on below my waist. He is a very honest, excellent physician who is secure enough to tell me he isn't equipped to tinker with my hormones. He recommends an associate of his, a gynecologist.

I dread the idea of spreading my legs and talking about my vagina and my sex life to a new doctor, so I put off calling for a month. When I finally call Dr. Matz's associate I am informed that he is ill. His office refers me to *his* associate. I make an appointment with Dr. Matz's associate's associate.

You can tell a lot about a doctor's practice just by looking at the magazines he has in his waiting room. This gynecologist had *Parents Magazine*, *Family Circle*, *McCall's*, and *Fortune*. No *Lear's* or *Modern Maturity*. This could only mean that his practice consists mainly of young mothers and that he's expensive, not the perfect doctor to see for menopause.

One of his many nurses escorts me to a small room, instructs me to remove all my clothing and put on a paper gown with the opening in the front. "The doctor will be with you shortly," the nurse says as she closes the door behind her. Twenty-five anxiety-filled minutes later, the doctor appears.

The gynecologist is about forty, neatly dressed, with a boyish face and huge manual-labor-type hands. As we exchange pleasantries he snaps on rubber gloves, rips open the autoclave bag, and pulls out a shiny speculum. He warms it in his huge hands, butters it with K-Y Jelly, and puts it in me like I'm a toaster oven.

I ride bareback in the cold metal stirrups as he peers into my vagina dispassionately giving me the facts: uterus smaller than normal, vaginal walls thin and fragile, minimal secretions, glistening appearance gone. He's talking about my insides like he's some kind of building inspector. What am I going to do about my thinning vaginal walls? Replaster? Spackle? "No, estrogen," he says. I am now completely hysterical. I am having an out-of-body experience. I imagine those old thinning walls in my vagina with a fresh new coat of estrogen. I hope it comes in decorator colors so that it won't clash with my old smaller-than-normal uterus. I feel like I'm an episode of "This Old House" and I want to switch channels.

He tells me I'm menopausal. I know it but I don't want to hear it. I say the word menopause. It comes out very tentatively. Now that it refers to me I hate the sound of it. For the first time I'm taking this menopause thing very personally. I tell him I don't want to take estrogen. It causes cancer. He tells me it's nothing to worry about. Sure. He's not taking it.

"Isn't there anything else?" I ask. He tells me there's Clonidine, a drug normally used for hypertension, and there are also Bellergal tablets for relief of the hot flashes, but it contains phenobarbital, a barbiturate sedative. No thank you. I'd rather keep the hot flashes and be able to operate heavy machinery. Next he tells me to gain some weight because heavier women tend to have fewer and milder hot flashes. I tell him I'm not doing it because heavier women also tend to have fewer and milder romances. He is not amused. He tells me how lucky I am and then rattles off in machine-gun fashion a list of menopausal ailments I could have had, stuff like weird dreams, lower-back pain, itching of the vulva, bouts of bloat, flatulence, indigestion, gas, rogue chin whiskers, aching an-kles, knees, wrists or shoulders, sore heels, thinning scalp, frequent urination, urinary leakage, swollen veins, light-headedness, dizzy spells, vertigo, panic attacks, cys-titis, depression, migraine headaches, crawly skin, and memory lapses. I tell him I wish I had the memory lapses so I could forget about all of this. Again, he is not amused. He has had enough of me.

As he ushers me out of his office he says, "You'll just have to learn to live with it." He must have studied at the Vince Lombardi School of Gynecology.

When I leave his office I am angry, depressed, and defensive. What does some young male gynecologist know about vaginas? He doesn't even own one. I blame the doctor but it's not his fault, it's mine. I was not pre-pared for the visit. I hadn't done my homework. I didn't ask the right questions. In fact I hardly asked any ques-tions. A doctor is only as good as his patient and I was a lousy patient.

Menopause was the biggest thing to hit my body since puberty and I was not prepared. What do you do when you outlive your ovaries? Wear black underwear at half mast? Say Kaddish? Light Tampax votive candles? No. What you do is assemble a team of friends, family, and doctors to help get you through it in the safest, most positive way.

Finding the right doctor is not easy. It takes trial and

error and a lot of work. Most women pick their doctor with less care than they pick a melon, and pound for pound there are probably more rotten doctors than rotten melons. If I had shopped as carefully for a gynecologist as I do for a cantaloupe I could have avoided a lot of bad situations. When your hormones are beating you up you need a doctor who has compassion and understands. Many don't. I have learned that there are three basic types of gynecologists to avoid: the Coach, the General, and the Mechanic. You already met the Coach—he was the one who attended the Vince Lombardi School of Gynecology.

The General has attended the Stormin' Norman Schwarzkopf School of Gynecology. He swaggers in with a starched white uniform, grunts a greeting, thrusts the speculum into your privates, snaps orders, barks commands, and totally intimidates you. He condescendingly tells you what's wrong and then maps out what "we" must do to attack the problem. It is your duty to follow the General's orders if "we" are to win Operation Desert Vagina. Not wanting to be among the few and the proud in the General's practice I immediately transferred out of his unit and signed on with the Mechanic.

The Mechanic has attended the Lee Iacocca School of Gynecology. His office is less like an examining room and more like an automotive diagnostic service center. I sit naked under a paper gown in one of his four or five little white service bays as he goes from patient to patient, bay to bay, examining our obsolete, overheated, out-of-tune vaginas. He has no emotion, no sense of humor, no personal touch as he moves along his menopause assembly line. He has no time to ask you how you are feeling. His high-tech machines and his tests will tell him. They tell him my endocrine system is shifting gears. He wants to fill my crank case with estrogen. I tell him the pit stop ends here and I'm going to get a second opinion from my local garage.

What I was looking for was a gynecologist who had a heart and a soul, someone who was interested in me and who cared about what I had to say. It's not easy spreading your legs and talking about your sex life and burning and itching and dryness to a doctor who treats you like a work order or a military operation. These bad experiences taught me what to expect from a good doctor and, more importantly, how to spot one.

You cannot judge a doctor by his address, the size of his office, or the number of laminated diplomas he has lining his walls. Good doctors are good because of certain qualities they possess that have nothing to do with the school they went to.

A doctor who is quick to pull out a prescription pad without considering nondrug remedies, or who relies heavily on machines, is not my kind of doctor. These time-saving, money-making techniques may be great for him but they mean nothing to me. I want him to spend his time listening to my complaints and symptoms, not some fancy computer.

The tests he orders are not half as important as how much he cares about you. I'm not talking about a love affair or a card on your birthday. I'm talking about remembering your name after the third visit and knowing your medical history before prescribing hormone replacement therapy. To me, attitude is as important as ability. I don't think a doctor is very smart when he makes you wait for an hour and then gives you five minutes. I think it's bad medicine to overbook your patients the way an airline overbooks passengers. This is the same doctor who takes your blood pressure and tells you it's high. Of course it's high. His would be high, too, if he had to wait an hour! If he can't give you his time don't give him yours.

I want my doctor to ask me what I eat and what vitamins I am taking. What we eat has a lot to do with how we feel, and yet most physicians don't know anything about nutrition. They are taught surgery in med school, not nutrition. The only thing they know about food is carving, cutting, and slicing. If they knew more about nutrition there probably would be less surgery.

I want my doctor to be patient, to understand, to listen. I don't want him to interrupt, cut the conversation short, split his attention between me, the patient down the hall, and the clock on the wall. I want him to not lie to me, to admit his limitations, to be secure enough to say "I don't know." I want him to make decisions *with* me, not for me, and I want him to be human. He is not God.

Because he is not God I no longer approach him in a state of awe. When I was a little girl my mother told me that doctors were special people and if I were lucky I would get to marry one. Times have changed and so has my attitude. Whenever I start doctor-worshiping all I have to do is remember some of those little creeps in high school who went on to med school and I am quickly returned to my senses.

I am no longer intimidated and insecure around doctors. If you have done your homework you know your body better than anyone does. And I always ask a lot of questions, especially if a doctor suggests hormones or any other kind of medication. This stuff isn't exactly bubble gum and I want to know what I'm getting into. I usually carry this list of questions with me:

- How does the medication work?
- What are the potential side effects?
- How safe is it?
- How long will I have to take it?
- What does it cost?
- Are the effects of the medication permanent?
- Different ways to take medication—pill, patch, cream?

- What is best for me?
- When should I take it? Should I take it with food?
- How long before it starts working?
- Can it be taken with other medications?
- Contraindications?
- What are the risks? What are the benefits?

And if I don't understand the answer, I ask again. Doctors can't write readable prescriptions. Why should we expect them to talk clearly?

After you've been through the diagnosis and the prognosis you still don't have to follow the doctor's orders, even if he or she tells you that a certain treatment is "indicated" or "necessary" or "the treatment of choice." Most of the tests in medical school are multiple choice, so his chances of the proper diagnosis are at best sometimes or never. Never always. And just because your gynecologist is a woman doesn't mean she is going to know more or be more understanding. Women go to the same schools as men and at present none teach courses in the power of positive menopause.

It is your body and your life and your money. Take charge. Choose a doctor who shares your values. If he's an action-oriented Coach or General or Mechanic, all for hormone replacement therapy or hysterectomy and you're not sure, see someone else. Don't worry about hurting his feelings. Worry about hurting yours. My father-in-law was told by his cardiologist that if he didn't have a triple bypass heart operation immediately he would die. That was ten years ago. Today, he is doing just fine. He never felt better. He never had the operation and never saw the cardiologist again. Sometimes an option is doing nothing. Fortunately, menopause is seldom fatal.

To most gynecologists the menopausal woman is not the most appealing of patients. To them the treatment of menopause has the excitement, the romance, and the glamour of hemorrhoids. They would much prefer delivering babies. It is positive, it is lucrative, and it is a growth industry. Menopause only interests them when there is surgery involved. Doctors are operators. The United States has the highest hysterectomy rate in the world. One out of every three women in the country will part with her uterus before she reaches the age of sixty. The conventional wisdom among gynecologists holds that when ovaries and uteruses are no longer needed for reproduction it is a good idea to remove them. Eight out of ten gynecologists are men. I wonder if they would be in such a hurry to remove the penis when it is no longer needed for reproduction. And if a doctor tells you he would recommend a hysterectomy for his own wife, find out more about their relationship.

THREE

Change-of-Life Beauty Queen

It was time to fit menopause into my life. To stop crying over spilled hormones and to start dealing with the lack of them. Estrogen was my body's freon and my cooling system didn't work without it, but I wasn't ready for hormone replacement therapy. Menopause is a natural process and I was determined to deal with it naturally and alone. No reason to call my mother. She has trouble dealing with these things. When I was ten she took me next door and had our neighbor Gertrude teach me the facts of life. Even if I did call her, I doubt if she would remember Gertrude's phone number. No need to talk to my father. He wouldn't understand. He still thinks of me as his baby, his little girl. In the windmills of his mind, a little girl, particularly his forty-seven-year-old little girl, is much too young for menopause. No need to alarm my husband with the news that his once-blushing bride is now flushing. He is having his own problems with mid-life. It was just going to be me and the night and the menopause.

It was not easy keeping the frequent and unpredict-able hot flashes from my husband. Anytime, anywhere, anyplace, I could be caught in the act of being menopaus-al. We could be sitting in the kitchen when the steam from a simple little hot cup of coffee would start me percolating. To cool down, I would get up, casually walk to our refrigerator, open the freezer door, and lean in. I would stay there until the flash passed or until my hus-band got curious. When he'd ask, "Are you out of some-thing?" I would mutter, "Yeah, estrogen," close the freezer door and pretend nothing happened. When we ate out, we ate out. The choice was always al fresco. To my husband it was romantic. To me it was pragmatic.

Unfortunately, in the bedroom, we did not sleep al fresco and there was no freezer to put my hot flashes in. Here I had to depend on my husband's sound sleep and my sound judgment in dealing with the fire and water. I would prepare for bed by hiding a large sponge and a change of clothes in my pillow, and two liters of water and a cordless fan under my side of the bed. But I was dreaming. No matter how much I prepared, the evening always wound up the same way. In the middle of the night I'd be nude, soaking wet, and red-hot on a soggy sheet. Next to me is my husband, in pajamas and a flannel robe, under the covers. He is in Anchorage and I am in Antigua. He is sleeping soundly. I am wide awake. When he awakes he asks me what's wrong. I tell him, "Too much coffee." I get up and put on a robe. It sticks to my damp body. When he asks why, I tell him it's static cling.

When a tide line appeared on the mattress I stopped buying my night clothes at Victoria's Secret and started buying them at the Foot Locker. I replaced my silky, sexy, nonporous things with heavy-duty sweat-absorbent gym clothes. Cotton became the fabric of my night life. I was now dressing in layers and wearing sweat suits to bed. What next, a wet suit? I was changing right under my husband's nose and he never said a word. How could he not know what was going on?

When I dusted I noticed that I wasn't just picking up dust, I was picking up hair. A lot of hair. My hair. I was shedding like a Shetland pony. My hirsute confetti was everywhere. It was obvious that my husband had also noticed the fallen hair. He never mentioned it, but every morning I would catch him checking his scalp in the bathroom with a hand mirror. I really felt bad not telling him what was going on, but if he was preoccupied with his male-pattern baldness he would be less aware of his flashing, shedding, menopausal wife. It was all getting out of control. My life was turning into some cheap horror movie. It was *Invasion of the Hormone Snatchers*, *The Night of the Living Hot Flashes*, and *Menopause from Hell.* Only it wasn't a movie, it was real, and I was the star. I had to talk to someone. It was time for other voices, other wombs.

Rita is my age, happily married, and a very good friend. In the past we have discussed infidelity, incest, rape, necrophilia, pedophilia, and everything else we had seen on "A Current Affair" and "Geraldo." We have revealed our deepest fears and anxieties. She has seen me at my worst. I have seen her at her most vulnerable. We have commiserated on everything from bad haircuts to spoiled children. When her kids were teenagers I sat with her as she worried that they were too dependent and would never leave. When they got older I sat with her as she worried that they were too independent and would leave. When they left we cried together as we assessed the damage to her wrecked parenthood. Over the years, we have discussed, argued, commiserated, quibbled, squabbled, and sympathized over pretty much everything except menopause.

Rita lives in Beverly Hills, the land of the rich, the skinny, and the young. It is not a place for menopause. Menopause means over the hill and you don't want to be over the hill in Beverly Hills. The life-style demands the right car, the right house, the right clothes, and, of course, the right condition. It is okay to have the latest fad disease like Epstein-Barr or even something terminal. It is not okay to have menopause. In Beverly Hills it is better to die young than to die of embarrassment.

In the few months since her kids left, Rita hasn't been feeling very well. She has been to gynecologists, dermatologists, proctologists, neurologists, and urologists. Her latest ologist, a rheumatologist, tells her he thinks she has lupus. She has all the symptoms—hair loss, fatigue, and aching joints. It will take awhile before he can make a definite diagnosis, so until then she cannot officially claim the disease as her own. I am not Miss Marple, the medical detective, and this is not an episode of "Menopause, She Wrote," but from her symptoms and my recent experience it seems clear to me that Rita has menopause, not lupus.

When in the most indirect, roundabout, subtle, sensitive, casual, nonthreatening way I suggest that maybe she might be experiencing some symptoms of menopause, Rita cuts me off at the pause. "Menopause?!!! Are you crazy? I'm too young. Do I look like Edith Bunker?!!!" Rita has never reacted this defensively or this violently to anything I have ever said or done. Obviously, I have pushed all the wrong buttons and have shorted her out. I try to recover by telling her I have the same symptoms as she and I have menopause. The second I say it, I'm sorry I said it. Rita is beside herself. She tells me I'm too young and I don't know what I'm talking about and that I should get another opinion. She also suggests that I take some more tests, including a polygraph.

I tell Rita that you don't have to be the Surgeon-General to know that we have menopause. It's no use.

She distances herself from me like it's contagious and I'm Menopause Mary. She just can't face the fact that her children and her youth have left her, and now her body is out of control, too. When I drop the subject we are both relieved. For some reason I was expecting her to have a relatively healthy attitude about menopause and not be so defensive. I, of all people, should have known better. And as a friend I should have been more sensitive to her feelings. I would have been plenty defensive if someone, even a good friend, had accused me of aging, especially if I lived in Beverly Hills, where menopause is grounds for divorce.

When I leave Rita I hate myself for my lack of sensitivity. I acted like I was a messenger from God. The Holy Gayle. Our Lady of a Thousand Hot Flashes. The truth is I am just like Rita. Just another woman having a tough time coming to terms with menopause. I needed another perspective.

There are several men in my life whom I consider part of my support system. No matter what happens they are always there for me. They are like my big brothers. My husband knows them and likes them. Whenever I had relationship problems or work problems or parent problems or whatever, I could talk to Lenny or Jack or Paul and they would commiserate with me. They had always been sensitive and understanding—that is, until I tried talking to them about menopause.

Jack is a fifty-eight-year-old bachelor who likes young women. The combined age of all his current dates is less than that of a single menopausal woman. When I ask Jack who his idea of a menopausal woman is he says Gloria Swanson in *Sunset Boulevard*. When I ask him to name a living menopausal woman he says Zsa Zsa Gabor. When I ask Jack what he knows about menopause he tells me about his mother's "changes." She spent a lot of time in a housecoat, in her dark stuffy bedroom, lying in bed with cold compresses. When I ask how old she was he tells me fifty-something. Very soon I will be fifty-something. Jack knows my age and for some reason he can't put me and menopause together. When I ask him how long before I hit menopause, he tells me fifteen years. According to his calculations my ovaries and I will retire at sixty-five. This is coming from an intelligent man with eight years of college and with degrees in science and engineering. Is this the new math?

Paul, a big lovable bear of a guy, is a successful stockbroker. He is Jack's age. He has been married three times and has divorced each woman before they reached menopause. Paul knows alimony, not menopause. When I ask Paul what he knows about menopause he tells me about college friends of his who would come home from working at a summer resort with stories of wild, older, hormones-out-of-control women chasing them around, trying to get these poor defenseless guys into bed. I am skeptical. Paul is a believer. "These guys had no reason to lie. They were all solid guys. All med students." Based on my recent experience, I bet most of them became gynecologists. When I ask him if he knew how old these wild women were he says, "Old. Forty-five, fifty." I drop the subject.

When I ask my friend Lenny what he knows about menopause he tells me the same red-hot menopausal mama story as Paul. Apparently the Insatiable Hot Menopausal Mama is right up there with other modern myths like the Loch Ness Monster and the Abominable Snowman—numerous sightings, specious reports, and very little concrete evidence. That is the way I would sum up most men's understanding of menopause. They have a genetic handicap. They just can't relate to the concept.

I have run out of friends that I can comfortably confide in and I feel alone and isolated. The hot flashes are still keeping me up most of the night. I toss and turn and toss and turn and toss and turn on the TV. I watch the late night movies on the all-Spanish TV channel thinking that maybe I can learn a second language. When the movies are over I switch to the Weather Channel and compare my hot, wet, sticky climate to the rest of the country's. Death Valley is sometimes hotter but I am always wetter. I then take inventory of my sweats, do a wash, and before I know it, it is 6:30 A.M., time to get up. I am up. I am Cranky, Sleepy, Achy, Itchy, Shaky,

Sweaty, and Crazy. I am Snow White and the Seven Menopausal Dwarfs. I look in the mirror. I do not see Snow White. I see the Seven Dwarfs. I ask them, "What have you done with Gayle?"

Late one night while lying in bed I heard a voice. It talked to me about menopause. It was one of those all-talk radio stations. The radio doctor was on the phone with a forty-nine-year-old woman who was having four hot flashes an hour, vaginal dryness, and had a family history of osteoporosis. For the hot flashes he recommended 800 I.U. (International Units) of vitamin E daily. For the vaginal dryness he suggested K-Y Jelly and having as much sex as possible: "If you don't use it, you'll lose it." For osteoporosis he recommended walking, climbing steps, and any weight-bearing exercise. When she asked him about HRT (hormone replacement therapy) he went crazy. He didn't believe there was enough evidence to prove it safe and he didn't know a single doctor who prescribed it for his wife. I wanted to know more about HRT but he was already on to ear infections. I called but I couldn't get through. It was busy. I called again. Busy. He is now talking about impotence. I hang up and redial for another twenty minutes. The line is busy. I keep dialing. Still busy. The show is over and I'm listening to a dial tone. If this were a medical emergency I would now be dead.

I have to find out more about hormone replacement

therapy. I have to get a second opinion. I try calling another radio doctor, a daytime radio doctor. Again, I cannot get through. He talks about corns and hiatus hernias and Retin-A, but no menopause. The next day I try calling before the show goes on the air. Busy. I press redial all the while the show is on the air. Still busy. When I finally get through the show is over and there is no answer. Maybe I should call 911.

Several days later, a menopausal woman gets through. It is not me. She is fifty-one, having mood swings, sleep disturbance, and urinary incontinence. The daytime radio doctor suggests estrogen. When she tells him that her family has a history of gall bladder trouble and hypertension he recommends the transdermal estrogen patch instead of the pill. It allows the estrogen to go directly into the bloodstream without first passing through the liver, thereby avoiding most of the reasons why some women can't take estrogen orally. This doctor is definitely in favor of estrogen and HRT. He says that women live a third of their lives after menopause and that estrogen can make the difference between a good life or simply existing. I must talk to this doctor and ask him if HRT is for me but again I can't get through.

I never get through. I am afraid I will never get a chance to turn down my volume. I have lost my patience and he has lost a patient. It is time to reach out and touch a live doctor again. I hope this time I can get through to him.

The phone rings. It is my friend Linda. She tells me she has been trying to reach me for days, but all she got was a busy signal. I'm so embarrassed. I tell her a lot of people have had trouble getting through to me lately. It is her fortieth birthday. To celebrate we decide to meet for lunch at one of those pretentiously understated places where people who "do lunch" lunch. I am excited. It will do me good to get out of myself and have some laughs. I hope the restaurant has good food and great air-conditioning. When I see Linda I don't have to ask her how it feels to be forty. She is borderline hysterical.

Tearfully, she hands me a birthday card. It is from her parents. The card is pretty much your standard overly sentimental parents-to-loving-daughter variety. Pink flowers under a syrupy verse filled with gooey synonyms for affection that rhyme with sappy words like dear and rare. On the back is a handwritten message from her parents. It wishes Linda the best of everything including a husband and children. The words husband and children are underlined.

I tell her that she shouldn't be so surprised and upset. That they didn't mean anything by it. Face it, most parents have an ancestor obsession. It's genetic. They think if they don't remind you, you'll forget. "Linda dear, when you're out get us a quart of milk, a loaf of bread, a son-in-law, and some grandchildren." Right now they are probably sitting at home pleased with themselves and their thoughtfulness. They're thinking they made your day and they can't wait for you to call and tell them the joy their special little message brought you.

Linda nods in agreement. "It's just that I'm forty and I don't need my parents to remind me that I'm not married and I'm not pregnant. They have been asking me for grandchildren since puberty. I get the message and I'm trying. It's just that everything I like is either illegal, immoral, or married."

Linda is a career woman. She has an exciting job in advertising production, with a lot of responsibility, and she makes a lot of money. But she would trade it in a minute for a decent guy and a kid. "I'm not exactly dateless and desperate, but time is running out. I'm forty, I am not in a relationship, my parents are on my back, I can hear that biological clock ticking loud and clear, and I'm scared. I don't even need a husband or a commitment. I could handle being a single parent. It's not that I want to retire to the country and raise children. I just want the opportunity to have a child. I want to be an ancestor, too." I try to comfort her by telling her she is only forty and has some time. She tells me that ten or fifteen years isn't such a long time. Because it is her birthday and she is not exactly having a good day, I don't tell her that if she thinks she has fifteen years she is dreaming. Linda knows about production, not reproduction.

When Linda asks me when my husband and I are going to have children I tell her I don't know. I don't have the stomach to tell her that I'm menopausal and can't have children. She knows I'm in my late forties. Right now it would be too depressing for her to hear and for me to talk about. When the waiter arrives with our food, neither of us feels much like chewing or swallowing, much less talking. We end the whining and dining with a piece of Black Forest chocolate cake and have it served with a flashing sparkler.

After lunch, I am starving for a child. The fact that I absolutely, positively can't have children has just sunk in and I feel an emptiness in my stomach. Until now I didn't think about it, not because it wasn't important. I didn't think about it because it was too important and too painful and too late. There was nothing I could do about it. Menopause is the ultimate birth control. The ball was over, the clock had struck twelve, and my reproductive system had turned into a pumpkin. Linda had it figured out and I didn't. When I was forty I wasn't preoccupied with kids. I was just preoccupied, thought I had plenty of time, no need to play "Beat the Clock." It was always too soon. Now it's too late. I wish I had consciously dealt with it or even stumbled into it. I wish it were kids that had changed my life, not menopause. The missed period used to mean I could be pregnant. Now it means I can't get pregnant. Same anxiety, different results. The pain of not giving birth is as painful as the pain of birth and it lasts a lot longer.

I feel like I have just lost an important job. That I have been given the pink slip, sacked, booted, bounced, and terminated. There will be no more periods. No more fertility. No children. I am washed up as a mother. Time to clean out my drawers, trash my Tampax, hand in my birth control, and punch out on the biological clock. It all happened so fast and without any warning. I feel angry and confused and betrayed. All I want to do is get home. Get into bed, pull the covers over my head, and stay there until this passes. The only problem is that menopause is not a pause. It is a full stop. Oscar Wilde wrote, "In this world there are only two tragedies. One is not getting what one wants and the other is getting it." He must have been talking about menstruation and menopause.

Now every time I see a pregnant woman I get mourning sickness. This is the birth of the blues. I hit the bookstore again. I am tempted by but bypass *Final Exit*, the last self-help book you'll ever need, in favor of a feel-good book called *14,000 Things to Be Happy About*. As you would expect, menopause isn't one of them. To help me come to terms with my new sense of vulnerability, mortality, and loss I even try reading some of those pop psychology books. Maybe, using their proven techniques, I can turn menopause into an opportunity. I read and read, trying to find ways to make the most of my menopause, to make menopause work for me. The results aren't very long-lasting. These books are like Chinese food. You read one and five minutes later you have to read it again.

Through it all the flashes continue. Every day on TV I watch Red Adair and his crew routinely put out another Kuwaiti oil well fire and I can't even stop a hot flash. Surely there must be some power that lies deep within me that will be my answer to Red Adair. To tap this power I try visualization.

"Thoughts are things," they told me in a seminar. All I had to do was create images and pictures in my mind that would put out the hot flash. Every time I felt a flash coming I visualized myself as an ice cube. Unfortunately, the ice cube always melted. At the second seminar they told me I needed a stronger image than a puny ice cube: "You can't stop a tank with a rock." And I also needed an affirmation. Affirmations are powerful positive statements encapsulating the ways in which we want to think, feel, and believe. I worked very hard on my visualizations and my affirmations, perfecting both the images and the words. Armed with my new and improved deterrent I was ready to once again do battle with the dreaded hot flash.

When I felt a flash coming I would now set these powerful images in motion. I would try to get comfortable and relax my body by breathing slowly and deeply from my belly. I would count down slowly from ten to one, feeling more completely relaxed with each count. Then in my mind I'd produce what was basically a one-minute beer commercial. I was a frosty can of beer embedded in a keg of ice, next to an igloo at the North Pole. Keeping these sharp powerful images in mind I would recite my affirmation. "I am frozen tundra. I am the polar ice cap. I am the Arctic Circle. I am glacial. I am ice." It was no contest. After a week the score was: hot flashes 175, visualization 0. Unfortunately, for me, visualization and affirmation weren't exactly the Patriot missile.

My only companion through the hot flashes and the night sweats and the insomnia was all-night television. The world of nocturnal TV is filled with miracles and miracle products. As you click your remote tuner you see entire programs devoted to molecular hair rollers, jet-stream ovens, brain superchargers, hair-cutting vacuums, and time-release breath mints. Powerful, charismatic miracle workers help you make money while you sleep, harness your alpha waves, and take control of your cellulite. In this world there is something for everything—nothing for menopause.

What we really need is a menopause channel on cable from midnight to 6:00 A.M. There are more than 40 million women going through menopause and a lot of us are up and flashing at this hour. Add another 20 million midlife crisis male insomniacs and you have a potential nocturnal viewing audience of 60 million viewers with good jobs and plenty of disposable income. We have the SportsChannel, the Weather Channel, and the Family Channel. Why not the Menopause and Midlife Channel? Program features could include hot-flash weather reports, biological clock time checks, midlife crisis talk shows, and my personal favorite, "Gayle's All-Night Menopause Pajama Party" with my special guests: Dyan Cannon, fifty-four; Ali McGraw, fifty-two; Ann-Margret, fifty; Marlo Thomas, forty-eight; and Goldie Hawn, forty-six. We could sell a lot of Os-Cal, Lubrin, Premarin, Replens, and other menopause accessories not available in stores. The M & M Network: Think of the possibilities.

I am tempted to write a letter to my midlife heroes, Ted Turner and Jane Fonda. They are both in their fifties but look like they're really hot for each other. I bet Ted and Jane still park and neck. I am jealous. Lately, my sex drive has gone from neutral to reverse, and with good reason. My vagina is dry, my clothes are wet, my hormones are low, and sex hurts. When my husband and I make love it feels like root canal. I moan like Monica Seles, but it is out of agony, not ecstasy. I scream "More!" praying he's had enough. He hadn't, but I had.

When I wake up one morning after a particularly bad seven-flash night looking like I've been through a car wash, my husband asks me if I'm coming down with something. "Yes," I tell him, "I'm coming down with

The Hot Tip

In the spirit of menopausal glasnost my husband encourages me to be open and honest with him. This new openness, while good for my head, does nothing for the rest of my body. I am falling apart faster than the Soviet Union. I begin sprouting rogue chin whiskers, develop an embarrassingly persistent itch between my legs, and find that the simple act of parallel parking causes my heart to shimmy and my body to overheat. In bed, the night sweats continue. Every night I hang on for dear life as I ride my raging hormones like a white-water rafter on a Sealy Posturepedic.

Unfortunately, I was taking my husband along for the ride. It was no longer my menopause—it was now our menopause. Every morning we would both get up wet and tired and cranky. My husband was getting contact menopause and it was rubbing him the wrong way. "All

I want is a dry bed and a good night's sleep, not a Rocky Mountain high. If I don't get some rest soon, I'm going to be camping in an oxygen tent.''

As the hormonal heat wave continues all my husband and I do is talk about my weather. We are obsessed with my highs, my lows, and my tropical depressions. We have become Mr. and Mrs. Willard Scott. The more I report the more we talk. But the nights remain wet and wild and the mornings continue to feel like the morning after. It is obvious that no amount of talking or caring or sharing is going to make it go away. The problem isn't in my head, it is in my uterus. If I don't see a gynecologist soon, we will both be needing a psychiatrist. It is time to get out from under my weather and get another second opinion.

A society friend of mine who menopauses in New York recommended her gynecologist, a world-renowned specialist in menopause. I called her. Unfortunately, she was not seeing new patients. She referred me to her protégé, Dr. Susan Brown. Based on my past experience I am leery of associates' associates, even if they are protégées. I make an appointment anyway.

Dr. Brown's waiting room is filled with pregnant women. Everyone is expecting and so am I. I am expecting to see more women my age. I see none. There is not a single menopausal patient or a single page of middle-age or menopausal reading material. I am sitting in the middle of another happy practice devoted to birth and babies. I feel as out of place as a fur coat at an animal rights convention. Are gynecologists specializing in menopausal patients extinct? I pick up a copy of *Parents Magazine* and hide behind it. There is a long wait. As I flip through an hour's worth of articles on "What to Name Baby," "Pickles and Ice Cream," "Cesarean Smarts," "Maternity Myths," "Building a Bassinet," and "Twenty-four Hours of Lamaze" I think about what I'm going to ask the doctor. This is not going to be like my last visit to a gynecologist. This time I have done my homework and I am much better prepared. I hope she is prepared for me.

Dr. Brown is a medical munchkin. She is small and round and close to the ground and around forty. I was expecting someone older, someone old enough to have actually experienced a hot flash. But hot flash experience aside, Dr. Brown is the kind of doctor you dream about. She is warm and caring and human—a real person, not some prescription dispensing medical vending machine. I feel very comfortable with her and give her my complete uncut and unexpurgated medical history. Dr. Brown patiently listens as I bitch about my every menopausal ache, itch, and twitch. She is in no rush. This is no pit stop. The only clock she is interested in is mine. Now I know why I had to wait an hour.

After the talking comes the testing. She has heard what I have to say. Now it is time to hear my body's side of the story. I get undressed, put on a gown, and am escorted to a room where a nurse gives me a complete blood analysis that includes liver and thyroid function, cholesterol and triglycerides and blood sugar levels and calcium and phosphorus levels. From there I move to the examining room for my pelvic exam and more surprises.

As I sit on the examining table I notice that the cold stirrups are covered with oven mittens and that Dr. Brown warms the speculum in a heating pad. It's not exactly Norman Rockwell or a fireside chat but it's a lot more welcome and cozy than any of my previous experiences. Dr. Brown begins by giving me a Pap smear and a vaginal smear to determine the presence of estrogen. She then gives me a breast exam and makes sure I know how to give myself a self-exam. When was the last time a doctor took the time to show you how to give yourself a breast exam? This doctor is too good to be true. A modern medical miracle. I am impressed.

Dr. Brown insists that I get a mammogram because the breast exam reveals that I have cystic breasts. This is not a surprise. I have heard it before. She says if I cut out all caffeine from my diet—coffee, tea, chocolate, soft drinks—in six months I will probably see a major reduction in the cysts. This is a surprise. I have not heard this before. Finally, a doctor who knows nutrition.

She also finds a benign fibroid tumor in my uterus

(little balls of muscle that form in the uterus in 20–40 percent of American women) and the start of a yeast infection that she tells me is common in menopausal women who are not on hormones. Cystic breasts, fibroid tumor, yeast infection. I have more things growing on me than a sunken ship. I thought menopause was supposed to be a time of growth, not growths. I get dressed and meet her in her office. It is bright and cheerful. I am not. She talks and I listen.

Dr. Brown tells me I'm no longer menopausal. It's been more than a year since my last period and now I'm officially postmenopausal. I haven't gotten used to the word menopausal and I've already been promoted to postmenopausal. In no other area I know of is advancement for women so rapid.

For my postmenopausal work she recommends HRT, or hormone replacement therapy, which is the combination of estrogen and progesterone, two hormones that the body produces naturally in the reproductive years. She says that the estrogen will control all my menopausal symptoms: the hot flashes, night sweats, vaginal dryness, and heart palpitations. It also provides protection from cardiovascular disease and the deadly bone-thinning disease osteoporosis. Heart disease is the number-one killer of women past the age of fifty and osteoporosis afflicts up to one-fourth of American women past the age of thirty-five.

Unfortunately, estrogen alone increases the chances of uterine cancer, so it must be taken with progestin (synthetic progesterone), which removes that risk. I will have to take one 0.625 mg tablet of Premarin (estrogen made from the urine of pregnant mares) every day from day one through day twenty-five. On day sixteen I add 10 mg of Provera (progestin) and also take it through day twenty-five. Then I am to stop taking both hormones for the remainder of the month. I start another cycle the first day of the next month.

There are some possible side effects from the combination of estrogen and progestin. Bloating, fluid retention, cramping, breast tenderness, nausea, and depression are not uncommon. "There will also be a continuation of menstrual bleeding," Dr. Brown adds. Pregnant pause.

"Could I still have a baby?" I say hopefully.

"I'm afraid not. It's just sloughing the uterine lining. You're not ovulating and you can't get pregnant." After she delivers the bad news there is another pregnant pause as the concept of blood without babies, and menopause with menstruation, sinks in. It is the ultimate curse. The thought of the two together is about as attractive as seasickness with lockjaw. I am relieved when she tells me that this side effect can be reduced or eliminated by altering the way progestin is given. Taking a lower dose of progestin (2.5 mg) every day of the month—instead of a stronger dose (5 mg or 10 mg) ten days a month—may make the periods lighter and after a few months may stop them altogether. The only drawback is that bleeding, if it does occur, is usually unpredictable, and since bleeding can be an early sign of uterine cancer she'd want to do uterine scraping to test for cancer if I were to bleed.

She is not finished. If I have liver disease, hypertension, high blood pressure, phlebitis (blood clots), gall bladder disease, obesity, or uterine fibroids, hormone replacement therapy might exaggerate the condition. I am now totally confused.

"You have just told me I have a fibroid tumor in my uterus and cystic breasts," I say. "I have read that estrogen causes breast cancer. Why on earth would you prescribe hormone replacement therapy?"

"If you have cystic breasts you're not necessarily at risk for breast cancer. Besides we'll be keeping a close watch on it with yearly mammograms and your monthly breast self-exams." Dr. Brown believes the benefits of HRT far outweigh the risks. Women on HRT tend to live longer, suffer fewer heart attacks, and have only one-half the risk of dying from coronary heart disease, which kills more women than all cancers combined and is the leading cause of death after menopause. It also prevents osteoporosis, eliminates hot flashes and other menopausal symptoms, improves your sex life, smoothes skin, tightens the bladder, firms breasts, increases muscle tone, and makes you feel better. Dr. Brown looks at me. "You are going to live more than a third of your life after menopause. Why not improve the quality of those years?"

All this information in one sitting is hard to swallow, impossible to digest, and very unsettling. It has gotten too complicated. Now it isn't just my menopause, now it's my cystic breasts and my fibroid tumor and my yeast infection and Premarin and Provera and bloating and cramping and bleeding and scraping and enough already. My plate is full. But we are not finished.

There are alternatives to taking HRT orally. The transdermal patch, which is worn like a Band-Aid, allows estrogen to enter the bloodstream directly without passing through the liver, thus avoiding the release of enzymes that could affect preexisting medical conditions. It is prescribed for people with liver problems, gall bladder disease, or hypertension. There is estrogen cream, which you use vaginally, but neither the cream nor the patch is as effective as HRT taken orally. The absorption of estrogen from the patch and from the vaginal cream varies so you can't be sure about the exact dose you are actually absorbing. And the cream is only basically effective for vaginal dryness and doesn't relieve severe hot flashes or prevent osteoporosis. Another option is progestin alone without estrogen. A daily dose of 2.5 mg of oral progestin can limit the frequency and severity of hot flashes. But that's all it can do. According to Dr. Brown, the only thing capable of handling the complete menopausal package is HRT taken orally.

I have been taking care of my body my whole life and as a reward for all this she is prescribing hormones. I don't believe in hormones. I have read what happens to chickens when they are fed hormones. The hens develop gigantic breasts and the roosters become capons. I am a free-range person. I don't eat anything that has chemicals, additives, or preservatives. I eat foods that have a shelf life, not a half-life. When the ingredients listed on the side of a package sound like they should be in a hand grenade I don't buy the product. If something's pickled, smoked, or cured I won't touch it. In my opinion, if it's cured it had to be sick to begin with. I refuse to turn my body into a chemical dumping ground filled with nitrites, nitrates, pesticides, dyes, waxes, and fumigants. If it's artificial, imitation, or synthetic I won't go near it. I am a natural person. Menopause is a natural process. It is not natural to put hormones made from the urine of a horse in my system. Any claims to the contrary, as far as I'm concerned, are pure horse manure.

I am not prepared to close shop, declare Chapter 11, and take Premarin and Provera for the rest of my now unnatural life. I ask Dr. Brown if there is anything natural I can take. She tells me vitamin E might work for my hot flashes: "Unlike other vitamins, it is not produced in the human body so I don't know why it works, but it can sometimes be very effective." If I want to give it a try I'm to start with 200 I.U. twice a day and if necessary to double the dose up to a daily total of 800 I.U. Under no circumstances am I to exceed 800 I.U. a day because any dose beyond that may interfere with the blood clotting mechanism. No prescription is necessary. I will give it a try.

For my vaginal dryness, Dr. Brown recommends a nonprescription, nonhormonal gel called Replens. It has few side effects and it has been approved by the FDA. Replens comes in single-use tampon dispensers, used every three days to provide continued lubrication. The gel helps normalize vaginal acidity and reduces the risk of infections.

As Dr. Brown tells me about the narrow and limited alternatives to HRT, she can sense that I am rapidly falling into a double-dip depression. She is very understanding. This is not the first time she has met with resistance. Only 20 percent of women who are given estrogen prescriptions actually fill them. She again tells me of her belief in HRT, especially for the prevention of osteoporosis, one of the most severe health problems that occurs in women. "One out of four postmenopausal women eventually suffers from serious osteoporosis and one-third of these women will die from complications of the disease." I definitely don't want to be a statistic. I ask again if it is safe. Dr. Brown again assures me that I am a perfect candidate for HRT. "I would definitely not recommend it if I suspected you had breast or uterine cancer, active liver disease, or blood clots, and I would hesitate if you had high blood pressure." I ask her if she would take HRT. "Absolutely." I believe in her. I also believe in Mother Nature. I believe I will make this decision myself. I need time. I have heard too much too fast. It is too soon to make a decision. The information is still whizzing by me at one hundred miles an hour. It has to slow down and sink in. We make a deal. I will take a bone-density test to determine if I have osteoporosis. If the test results show that I have no signs of osteoporosis I won't have to take HRT. I can live with that and I hope I will.

For now Dr. Brown does insist that I get 1,500 mg of calcium in my diet daily. "When there is not enough calcium available from the food you eat, your body will take what it needs right out of your bones," she says. She tells me about a new product called Calcimilk. It is calcium-fortified, lactose-reduced, and low-fat, and vitamins A and D are added. One eight-ounce glass has 500 mg of calcium. "The advantage of getting your calcium from food rather than from pills is the other nutrients that food has to offer." If I want to use a supplement she recommends calcium citrate. It is very well absorbed, usually doesn't cause either flatulence or constipation, and the risk of kidney stone formation is reduced. "Never take more than 600 mg at one time. Your body will not absorb more than that. Take it with your meals and at bedtime with eight ounces of water." Dr. Brown also gives me a typed list of calcium-rich foods with their exact calcium content in milligrams.* On the list I write "vitamin E" and "Replens" so I won't forget. I go home with a lot of respect for Dr. Brown, the telephone number of several hospitals that offer bone density testing, and a lot to think about.

To estrogen or not to estrogen: That is the question. It would be great to get a good night's sleep and a good night's sex and skin that looks younger and to feel better and not to worry about heart disease and osteoporosis. But is estrogen safe? True, the dosage is smaller than it used to be and with the addition of progestin there is no threat of uterine cancer, but estrogen is still linked to breast cancer and women over fifty account for about two-thirds the cases of breast cancer. Dr. Brown says my risk of breast cancer is small. Small is not good enough. It is my breast and it will be my cancer. I want no risk. Why do I have to trade freedom from heart disease and osteoporosis for a possible breast cancer? These are serious, deadly illnesses and I'm trading them like recipes. And even if I do trade how do I know that the use of progestin with estrogen won't cancel the benefits that

*See Notes for Dr. Brown's Calcium Content List.

estrogen alone offers for heart disease and osteoporosis? I have read that some doctors think it does. If I play my cards wrong I could wind up with all three. There is a history of breast cancer in my family and since I have no children I am even at greater risk. There is also a history of osteoporosis and cardiovascular disease. So it is a very difficult choice, especially since concrete information about the long-term effects of estrogen and progestin in combination won't be known for years. There is, however, plenty of solid information about estrogen.

Since its introduction in the late forties, estrogen has had more ups and downs than the hemline. It debuted as DES, a drug that was used to prevent miscarriage and "make a healthy pregnancy healthier." It was taken off the market after the discovery that it caused vaginal cancer and congenital abnormalities in children born to women receiving the drug in pregnancy. A short while later it came back in the birth control pill. After the pill was linked to breast cancer, blood clots, heart attacks, and liver and gall bladder diseases, they went back to the drawing board. In the sixties estrogen resurfaced as the wonder drug that would slow the aging process and make women "feminine forever." By 1975 it was one of the top five prescription drugs in the United States. But nothing is forever. It happened again. They found that it was now linked to gall bladder disease and uterine cancer. Estrogen has been hailed as a wonder drug. Based on its record, it's a wonder that it is still on the market.

If estrogen were prescribed for men instead of women and the drug had this same history, you can be sure it would have been exposed on "60 Minutes," discussed by the "McLaughlin Group," debated in the House, investigated by the Senate, and settled in the courts with the usual fine, jail, and community service.

The medical community believes the merger of estrogen with progestin is the new growth stock. They say the combination of the two best imitates the hormones of our menstrual cycle. I was hoping for a natural supplement, not a female impersonator. Saccharin was a fake sweetener that imitated sugar and caused real cancer of the bladder in laboratory animals. Why should I be bullish on estrogen and progestin? The progestin Provera has never been approved for treatment of menopause by the FDA. Why should I have confidence in this new therapy? It is from the same type folks who brought us DES, the Pill, breast implants, and Dalkon Shields. We have suffered more casualties from Dalkon Shields than Desert Shield and Desert Storm combined. This is serious stuff, yet virtually all the research is being done by men who know very little about women and almost nothing about the menopause experience. To help them better understand the effects of medication on women they first test it on rats. What do rats know about the modern woman? Rats don't get hot flashes and buy Tampax and wear bras and bring the car in for service and remember everyone's birthday. Rats can't cook and clean and shop and entertain. The only thing rats and the menopausal woman have in common is rogue chin whiskers. You can't learn a thing about women from rats. You learn about women from women. Human women are the only creatures on earth who experience menopause. That's why we are a generation of guinea pigs.

If we weren't guinea pigs why would they let us take estrogen and progestin in combination without exhaustive long-term testing? They say it works fine and there is nothing to worry about. They said the same thing when birth control pills were mass-marketed after only three years of observation on a mere 132 women. The Pill worked fine—except I read it caused breast cancer in some women, which was plenty to worry about. They say that progestin with estrogen eliminates the risk of uterine cancer. Maybe there are other, more serious risks and side effects that we don't know about. Hydrogen worked fine for dirigibles but the passengers on the *Hindenburg* couldn't live with the side effects. Don't get me wrong: I'm a big believer in things working in combination. It works great in the kitchen. Ketchup and mayonnaise make a great Russian dressing. But they are condiments, not hormones. If you mix estrogen and progestin the result might not be Russian dressing. It might be Russian roulette. They say that if I take HRT it will make menopause a memory. I just don't want it to make me a memory. Is estrogen and progestin ketchup and mayonnaise? Or hydrogen and dirigibles? Or am I comparing apples and oranges? It's all very confusing. I have been able to live without HRT. Can I live with it?

A Bone-Chilling Experience

I call to make an appointment for my bone-density test at one of the orthopedic hospitals in New York City. They schedule two appointments, one for the test and the other for a follow-up consultation.

In my mailbox, five days later, is a large envelope from the hospital. Enclosed is an appointment card, a medical questionnaire, and a risk profile. The medical questions are detailed but pretty standard. The risk profile is another story. It is anything but standard, particularly what I call the Un-American Activities Section, which asks questions with definite racial overtones. Am I black or white or Oriental or Catholic or Buddhist or Jewish? Am I Northern European or Eastern European or African? I get the feeling that this hospital is run by the Department of Immigration and Naturalization and the test is being administered by the FBI. If I don't do well I will be deported.

When I check in for the bone-density test at the

hospital I am directed to the Nuclear Medicine wing. Nuclear medicine is a fancy name for X-rays. Here I am greeted by an extremely hip, young, green-jacketed Latin technician. As he leads me to the X-ray room, he prepares me for the experience. He tells me that he will be using the single- and dual-photon scanners, which measure the wrist, forearm, spine, and hipbones in my body and can detect even the smallest change in my bone density. He goes on to say that the whole process takes only a couple of minutes and that the scanners use one-twentieth the radiation of a chest X-ray. I am sure that this has got to be exciting news for those diet-conscious patients who are counting roentgens. At last, a lite X-ray. I go into a tight little cubicle, slip into a loose-fitting green gown, and join a group of little old men in shoes and socks and gowns headed for the X-ray room.

The X-ray room is very much like my gown. It is large and green and cavernous. X-ray equipment hangs from the ceiling, rises from the floor, and extends from the walls. There are no windows. No need for windows. Here people look in, not out. The room is crackling with energy. Some of it is nuclear, most of it is from the radiologic technicians who buzz around the buzzing equipment posing patients, snapping pictures, and cracking X-rated inside roentgen jokes to their coworkers as their machines move forward, up and down, and in and out. These guys are pros. This definitely is not airport security. This is nuclear medicine.

My guy has his own style of working. He operates less like an X-ray technician and more like a high-fashion photographer. As far as he's concerned this is not an X-ray; this is a photo session. I share the fantasy. I am now Cindy Crawford and he is Scavullo. Scavullo positions me on a table and begins ordering and asking and posing and kidding and joking. "Over more. Higher. Lower. Hold your breath. Don't move. Relax. Great." Before I know it, I am on my back, legs up like a dog about to have its stomach rubbed with 95 percent less radiation than a chest X-ray. He presses a button and a large overhead machine slowly and silently passes over my landscape like a spy plane taking reconnaissance photos of my infrastructure.

Scavullo then leads me to a smaller machine where he takes extreme close-ups of my wrist. Throughout it all he is laughing and smiling. You can tell that he loves his work. I bet his X-rays are on the cover of all the nuclear medicine magazines. When the session is over I ask him when I will get the results. He tells me in two weeks. Scavullo would have had them tomorrow. But these are X-rays, not photos, and this is for osteoporosis, not *Vogue,* and I am not Cindy Crawford and he is not Scavullo. Reality is a bitch.

When you live in a world of instants two weeks is a long time to wait. I'm used to instant coffee, oatmeal, and even credit. There's microwave popcorn and quick-drying paint and faxes and Polaroids and next-day delivery anywhere in the world. You can even get hot pizza delivered to your door in thirty minutes or less, guaranteed or your money back. But I have to wait two weeks to find out if my bones have turned to grated Parmesan cheese. That's a long time but I can handle it. Besides, I am confident there is nothing to worry about.

When my mother calls I mention the bone-density test. To my surprise she knows all about it. "Nothing to it. The whole thing takes a few minutes." I ask her how she did. "I failed. They told me I had osteoporosis." I ask her why she didn't tell me. "What's to tell? You've got to expect those things at my age. Bones aren't Tupperware, they wear out after seventy years." Her not telling me is not unusual. We come from a long line of "keep it to yourselfers," the philosophy being, if you ignore it, it will go away. I ask her if she knew she had osteoporosis. "Of course not. There aren't any symptoms. You don't know you have it until you get it. Got it?" I get it. "Your aunt Martha, may she rest in peace, never took a test, always drank a lot of milk, said it was 'money in the bank.' She was a big healthy woman just like you, always felt great until she broke her hip, got shorter, and found out she had osteoporosis and didn't feel great anymore." We get off the subject of my aunt Martha and back to my mother. "They wanted me to take estrogen and told me to stop smoking and drinking coffee and to start exercising." I ask her what she did. "I bought a Jane Fonda tape." I'm about to tell her to stop smoking when she says, "And don't tell me to stop smoking, I can't." I don't. "And I gotta have my coffee, it keeps me regular."

There is a double standard here. This is a woman who for health reasons insisted that I never sit on a public toilet seat, never drink from someone else's glass—even a friend's, never take food from strangers, and get a tetanus shot after contact with anything rusty. I do not remind her of this. Instead I ask her if she considered taking estrogen. "I'd never take that stuff, not with my fibroid tumor. Besides, estrogen makes you bleed. In my lifetime I've had five hundred periods, give or take a couple. I don't want any more. Enough is enough. When you're seventy, you don't want to be schlepping around buying Tampax and going to doctors every five minutes for biopsies and Pap smears and consultations." I tell her an iron will and brittle bones are not a good combination. "If you keep this up you're going to be the Hunchback of Queens Boulevard." I can tell she is now very uncomfortable and doesn't want to talk about it anymore. We spend the rest of the call talking about fluid retention, something we are both comfortable with. I now add bones and disease to the birds and the bees and the already long list of other things I shouldn't talk to my mother about.

After I hang up, I get hung up on the idea that maybe I do have osteoporosis. My mother has it, my aunt Martha had it, I'm postmenopausal, I drink coffee and colas, and I never went out of my way to drink milk and take calcium. If I wasn't at risk Dr. Brown certainly wouldn't have insisted that I have a bone-density test and that I immediately begin taking calcium supplements. She didn't suggest, she insisted. My bones aren't telling me anything. Everybody else is. I look in the mirror. Staring back at me is me. I was expecting to see Whistler's mother. Unfortunately, it is not important what I see or think or feel. With osteoporosis instinct is inoperative. I won't know anything until I get the results of my bone-density test. I drown my sorrows in a quart of milk and go to bed.

In bed, I lie awake thinking about my aunt Martha and her "money in the bank," faithfully drinking her milk and making her calcium deposits, confident she was building strong bones that would last forever. Little did she know that osteoporosis, like some high-rolling, low-life swindler, had taken over and robbed her bones of her life savings of calcium and other minerals. When her bank collapsed there was nothing left but a crumbling skeletal system and a bunch of worthless junk bones. "Osteoporosis." Just saying the name gives me the creeps.

The next day my uneasiness over my shrinking skeleton grows from mild neurosis to full-blown osteopsychosis. This was triggered when I asked myself the question: "So, let's say you do have it. What's the worst that can happen?'' And the answer was: ''I could break my hip, develop a dowager's hump, be four foot nine, look six months pregnant, be bedridden, in constant pain, turn into an amoeba, and disappear from the face of the earth.''

My new fear of height and the loss of it triggers a major change in my eating habits. The calcium list that Dr. Brown gave me takes on a new importance. It is now my dietary bible. I study it very carefully. I find that dairy products have more milligrams of calcium than other food sources. I can get my daily requirement of 1,500 mg of calcium from five eight-ounce glasses of milk. That's a lot of milk, but it's a drop in the bucket when you compare it to some other sources of calcium. If you find it hard to digest milk or are allergic to dairy products, it's not so easy to get your 1,500 mg of calcium naturally. Vegetables and nuts—collards, broccoli, turnip greens, arugula, almonds—are a good source. But corn, bean sprouts, and cashew nuts aren't. You would have to eat three hundred ears of steamed corn or thirty-seven pounds of bean sprouts or twelve and one-half pounds of cashew nuts to get your daily requirement of 1,500 mg of calcium.

Canned salmon and sardines and mackerel are excellent sources of calcium. But not all fish are created equal. There are only 6 mg of calcium in a three-ounce can of tuna. That would mean that you would have to eat

250 three-ounce cans of tuna every day to meet the 1,500 mg daily requirement. That's like trying to suck a day's worth of coins out of a parking meter. If tuna is your only source of calcium you're in deep trouble. You're in even deeper trouble if you're a junk-food junkie. To get your 1,500 mg of calcium you would have to eat 132 glazed doughnuts, or 582 hot dogs, or 2,688 french fries every day. If you wash it all down with thirty-six quarts of beer you'll get another 1,500 mg of calcium.

It takes about six months for the next two weeks to pass. During this time I breakfast on broccoli, snack on sardines, drink milk from the container, and buy calcium citrate supplements. I also buy vitamin E for my hot flashes and Replens for my dry vagina. So far, the vitamin E gets an F for the prevention of hot flashes. They push the vitamin E aside and keep coming and coming and coming. The Replens is another story. When I try it, my dry vagina becomes covered with a long, stringy, cheese-like substance that looks like a canapé topping. I don't know what the stuff is but whatever it is, I bet it contains more calcium than a three-ounce can of tuna. Sex with Replens is definitely less painful but it makes me feel like I'm an hors d'oeuvre. You get one dozen Replens for $18—that's $1.50 per serving. A lot of money for an appetizer but a small price to pay for painless sex.

The day of my bone-density test consultation I get up at 6:00 A.M. The appointment is at noon. To make sure I get there on time I leave the house at 9:30 A.M. I am stuck for well over an hour in midtown traffic and I am still forty minutes early. I wait in a room with green plastered walls filled with outpatients in white plaster casts. As I sit next to these people nursing their broken bones I feel out of place and out of my mind. All I can think about are the results of my bone-density test. Will they find cheesecloth instead of bone? Will I wind up looking like the Leaning Tower of Pisa? I work myself up into a quiet frenzy and spend the next forty minutes dealing with woulda's, coulda's, and shoulda's.

When Elizabeth Treadwell, the director of the osteoporosis program, greets me in the waiting room, I am completely out of control. I don't even have the courtesy to say hello. The first words out of my mouth are, "Do I have osteoporosis?" She smiles warmly and leads me to her office. The room is small and the surroundings intense but she is relaxed and friendly and pretty. When we enter the office I ask again. She is not letting my neurosis get in the way of her agenda. She calmly opens my file, smiles broadly, and with great pleasure tells me that my test results were excellent. I am three percent above normal for my age group. When I hear the news I am not only relieved, I am exhilarated. I feel like I have just won the Publishers Clearing House Sweepstakes. I won't have to take estrogen. I can deal with my menopause naturally. I can relax. Hallelujah! I feel ten feet tall.

Wanting to put my score in perspective I ask her what a bad score would be. Bad is 20 percent below normal for your age group. At 50 percent below normal for your age group you have hit the "fracture threshold." Here the bone is weak enough for a simple fall to break it. Below this level you enter the House of Pain. Here a sneeze can result in a broken rib and lifting a Kleenex can mean a broken wrist. Assured that I am far away from my first fracture and that I am nowhere near downtown osteoporosis, we proceed with the consultation.

We begin by reviewing my risk profile. The fact that I am female, Caucasian, of Northern European ancestry, have smoked, am small-boned, have a family history of osteoporosis, exercised too much, was a vegetarian, drank diet colas and coffee, wasn't fat, and am currently postmenopausal will greatly affect my chances for getting osteoporosis. Huh? I doubt if even Sherlock Holmes could find the connection between any of this and brittle bones.

Elizabeth Treadwell, with the precise logic and British accent of a Scotland Yard chief inspector, explains that osteoporosis, like some deranged serial killer, does not strike randomly. "There are certain genetic, medical, and life-style factors that make some people more at risk than others. Just being a woman increases your risk of osteoporosis. Most of the 25 million advanced cases of osteoporosis are in women. It affects one in four women in the United States. For women the loss of bone begins sooner and proceeds six times more rapidly than it does in men. Our smaller frames may be the reason. When the body needs calcium and calls on the bones to give up some, men's bones simply have more to give." This is probably the only area where a man has a greater capacity to give than a woman and we have to pay with our bones. Osteoporosis is definitely not an equal opportunity destroyer.

It's tough being a woman, especially if you are a Caucasian or Oriental woman. Women whose ancestors come from Northern Europe, China, and Japan are at greater risk than black women. "Black women have larger muscle and skeletal mass and appear to lose bone at a slower rate than Caucasian women," Elizabeth says. Another clue as to whether or not you are at risk is genetic. If osteoporosis runs in your family there is a good chance it will be creeping into your bones. I take no comfort in the fact that my mother and my aunt, both Northern Europeans, have been visited by this silent deadly misogynist.

Not all risks are inherited. Some are acquired. When I told Elizabeth that I sit all day and write she reminded me that sitting all day builds wide buttocks, not strong bones. Weight-bearing exercise builds bone. Sitting is weight bearing but it definitely isn't exercise. "People who are bedridden and astronauts who are weightless in space rapidly lose bone mass no matter how much calcium they consume.'' If you have a sedentary life-style you are at risk. She emphasizes that "exercise like brisk walking and tennis and even weight lifting are essential to maintaining strong bones.'' The fact that I did aerobic dancing, jogged, and lifted weights almost every day put me at less risk.

Unfortunately, too much exercise can be as bad as too little. It can cause amenorrhea, which is the absence of a normal menstrual cycle for a prolonged period of time. When you have amenorrhea the amounts of estrogen and progesterone are drastically reduced, which leads to bone loss. This happened to me when I was thirty, during my "you can't be too rich or too thin period," which through too much hard work and too frequent and too intense exercise turned into my no-period period. It was all too much for me and I stopped immediately. According to Elizabeth Treadwell, if I hadn't cut down on the exercise and my period hadn't returned, I would now have the skeletal mass of an invertebrate.

As we continue to review my profile, I can see where I am headed and I don't like it. So far everything I did or didn't do in my life puts me at risk. After I got the results of the bone-density test I felt ten feet tall and confident. But with each new piece of information I feel less confident, much shorter, and at greater risk.

I had smoked for twelve years. Smoking increases a

person's risk of osteoporosis. The bone density of women who smoke is lower than that of women who don't, and menopause in smokers may occur one or two years earlier. The fact that I drink four cups of coffee and a couple of diet colas every day also doesn't help my cause. Elizabeth tells me, "We only lose about 11 mg of calcium per caffeinated beverage. If you drink no more than two or three cups a day no problem. The loss can be made up with a few swallows of milk." But she warns that if you drink ten or twenty cups a day, make another pot for osteoporosis. "If you want to keep calcium in your bones, reduce your intake of foods that are high in phosphorus and low in calcium." In other words, if you live on coffee, cigarettes, alcohol, diet cola, steak, and cake, followed by an antacid containing aluminum, you can kiss your bones good-bye.

The deeper we get into my risk profile the lower I feel. Every new risk factor reminds me of something I'd rather forget. When Elizabeth Treadwell tells me that it is suspected that pure vegetarians who don't eat dairy products have a hard time getting calcium and adequate protein, I casually mention that I was a vegetarian for about seven years. When she asks me what I ate during those years that I was "into health," I tell her vegetables and grains. Surely all those green vegetables and grains that I ate had to be loaded with bone-building calcium. They were. The only problem is that many of my favorites, like dandelion, asparagus, beet greens, Swiss chard, parsley, rhubarb, and spinach, not only contain calcium but also contain oxalic acid, which blocks the absorption of calcium in the body. "And the grains?" I ask desperately. She shakes her head sympathetically and reveals that phytic acid, which is found in many high-fiber foods such as grains, may interfere with the absorption of calcium.

As we unravel the mystery of osteoporosis I start to unravel and realize there is no mystery to osteoporosis. This is not a "who done it." We know who done it. The question is, Who is it going to do it to and what is going to be done about it? So far I am nine for nine on the osteoporosis hit list and I am nervous, very nervous. I am calmed by the fact that Elizabeth Treadwell is calm. If she isn't nervous there is no reason for me to be. I am sure the worst is over. It isn't.

More dangerous than my fair skin, my Northern European background, my family history, my small bones, my sedentary work habits, my soft drinks, coffee, vegetarianism, and amenorrhea is the fact that I am post-menopausal. Menopause takes the biggest toll of all on the skeletal system. Estrogen helps maintain bone mass and strength. When menopause shuts down the supply, more bone is lost and less is formed; the bones become thinner and are more susceptible to fractures. Women who experience menopause before the age of forty-five without the protection of hormone replacement therapy are at even greater risk.

I am overwhelmed by this latest bone-chilling news. I am now ten for ten and on my way to the Brittle Bones Jackpot—a lifetime supply of breaks, fractures, pain, and extended hospital stays. Is there any risk I don't have? Am I the perfect victim? Will I be next? I can no longer control myself. "Am I at high risk?" I ask casually.

She tells me that there is no evidence of bone loss and I am at moderate risk. I could be at much greater risk if I were a red-headed, blue-eyed, freckle-faced, alcohol-drinking, heavy-smoking, meat-eating, bedridden astronaut from Norway who had thyroid disease, scoliosis, and was on cortisone and aluminum-laced antacids. At greatest risk would be a menopausal astronaut with all the above-listed options. An unlikely occurrence. Elizabeth then tells me that no matter how many risk factors you have you still may not get osteoporosis. The only foolproof determination of osteoporosis is the bone-density test, and mine was negative. Then out of the blue, just when I think I am safe and can go home, she suggests that I take estrogen.

"Estrogen? You just told me that I did great on my bone-density test and I'm only at moderate risk. Why estrogen?" She explains, "We want to keep it that way. Estrogen is vital to the absorption of calcium and is essential to the maintenance of bone mass and strength. One out of four women lose bone rapidly during the first seven to ten years after menopause, and estrogen plays an important role in the prevention of postmenopausal bone loss. HRT starting at menopause and continuing for at least five to ten years reduces the risk of osteoporotic fractures by at least 50 percent to 60 percent, perhaps more." When I tell her about my deal with Dr. Brown and my reluctance to take hormones for menopause she sympathizes, but emphasizes, "I am not suggesting that you take it for your menopausal symptoms; I'm suggesting that you take it for the prevention of osteoporosis. Menopause is not a disease but osteoporosis definitely is. And a crippling one at that. If you don't take estrogen you are at risk and may lose more bone. It's that simple."

Gulp. I am absolutely, positively convinced that what she says is irrefutable but I am not prepared for this unpleasant little surprise. Less than ten minutes ago I thought I had won the Publishers Clearing House Sweepstakes; now she is suggesting I give back the prize and pay for the magazines. "Would you take estrogen?" I ask defensively. "I do," she says. Not would. Does. Sitting directly across from me is a woman who is currently under the influence of HRT and who is definitely enjoying the influence. I have a real good view of her and she looks real good. She is alive, vital, skin glowing, extremely sharp, alert, and patient. Obviously, she has had a dry bed and a good night's sleep. We are contemporaries, except she had worked it out and I was still finding out. "How do you like HRT?" I ask. You don't have to be a psychic to know the answer. She doesn't like it. She loves it.

"Besides its obvious health factors, women who take estrogen enjoy a better quality of life. It is speculated that it raises our endorphin levels, which are our natural pain relievers. Exercise also increases endorphins. When your endorphin levels are up you have more vigor and zest and a better sense of well-being." This woman is a true believer and I can see why.

Elizabeth Treadwell is not some out-of-control, born-again hormoner. She is a smart, sensible, responsible woman to whom the word "menopause" is not an abstract concept like heaven or hell. She has been there. She has actually felt the flush of the hot flash and the rush of the night sweat. She knows from experience what life was like before HRT and she knows what life is like after and she's telling me after is better. She had been through it and I could tell that she was really interested in helping me through it. You have to listen carefully to someone who practices what they preach.

"Do I have to start HRT immediately?" She tells me it will do me more good if taken early rather than late. "Estrogen is given to prevent rapid postmenopausal bone loss which occurs during the first seven to ten years after menopause. But it will do you some good no matter when you start." "Once I start, can I stop?" "If estrogen is stopped after seven to ten years there will be some bone loss (but you are still ahead of the game) and bone loss continues at a gradual rate. Estrogen cannot replace bone." I hear her loud and clear but I don't want to start something I can't stop. She's very understanding and we move on.

She tells me that they are testing a new "optimistic intervention" on menopausal women who are not taking estrogen for osteoporosis. It is a battery-operated electric corset that stimulates bone formation. They have used it successfully on complicated, slow-healing fractures. They believe it will help in preventing osteoporosis when used to stimulate spinal bone in menopausal women (the spine is where we suffer the most bone loss immediately following menopause). She asks me if I want to be in the study. The second she says this I have an image of little lab mice running around in little electric corsets. But that is not why I decline the offer.

I know the corset is battery-operated and I'm sure it is safe, but I am taking no chances. Electricity and water are a lethal combination and with the frequency and intensity of my night sweats, I am afraid of either shorting the equipment or dying of electrocution. I also share my bed with a husband who has been through enough wet nights to give him free-floating anxiety. At this point I doubt if he would appreciate the shock of the new, even if it is of extremely low voltage.

Since I wasn't going to take HRT or try the corset, our next goal was to find a way for me to get enough calcium to keep my bones healthy and strong. Ninety-nine percent of your body's calcium is stored in your teeth and bones. The remaining 1 percent is in your blood and soft tissue and is absolutely essential for your life and health. Without these normal blood calcium levels your muscles, including your heart muscles, wouldn't contract correctly. Your blood wouldn't clot and your nerves wouldn't carry messages. The body doesn't manufacture calcium, so when blood calcium levels fall, the body will immediately take whatever it needs from the body's cookie jar, the bones. Unless we can keep the bones supplied with enough calcium they will become weak and brittle.

To prevent the removal of calcium from bone it is essential that we get certain minimum amounts in our diet. Daily recommended calcium requirements range from 800 mg for adult men and women, to 1,500 mg for young adults aged twenty-five to thirty-five and for post-menopausal women like me. Elizabeth would recommend 1,000 mg if I were on HRT. Calcium-rich foods like dairy products, fish, shellfish, and dark green vegetables may not be enough. Calcium is hard to hang on to. Not all the calcium we take in is absorbed by the body. We may need to consume greater amounts of calcium just to get the minimum required for healthy bones. At best only 20 percent to 40 percent of the calcium we ingest is absorbed. Sometimes supplements are needed to get us the recommended daily allowance. Calcium carbonate and calcium citrate are the two most frequently recommended formulas. In choosing a supplement the key is the amount of elemental calcium. Elemental calcium is the actual calcium that is ingested by the body. Calcium carbonate has the highest concentration of elemental calcium: 40 percent. This means that a 600 mg tablet of calcium carbonate gives you 240 mg of elemental calcium. The higher the concentration the fewer pills we need to swallow. But no matter how many pills you swallow you can only absorb 600 mg of calcium at a time. And you shouldn't take more than 2,000 mg a day. Absorption is best in an acid environment, so the supplements should be taken just before a meal, when hydrochloric acid in the stomach is at an optimal level. Persons over seventy do not produce as much hydrochloric acid, so absorption in this situation is best after a meal. But most important is not when you take it but *that* you take it.

Unfortunately, there is no FDA regulation governing the manufacture of vitamins and minerals. Some brands of calcium carbonate tablets do not disintegrate quickly enough in the stomach to ensure absorption. Elizabeth gave me a little tip to help me pick out the winners from the losers, the good from the bad. If a calcium carbonate tablet does not dissolve into fine powder within half an hour when covered with white vinegar, it is probably not disintegrating rapidly enough in the stomach to ensure absorption (the acidity in the vinegar is similar to hydro-chloric acid in the stomach).

Calcium carbonate also has a couple of unappetizing side effects. It can cause constipation and flatulence. If you work in close quarters with a lot of other people and you want to keep your work environment friendly and cordial, I would not recommend it. Fortunately, calcium citrate is an excellent alternative. It is very well absorbed, regardless of the level of acidity, and does not cause either flatulence or gas. Because it is lower in the amount of concentrated or elemental calcium (24 percent), more tablets need to be taken. But I consider this a small price to pay for fresh air and dignity.

You can pop calcium supplements all day but it won't do you a bit of good unless it's absorbed by the body. Without vitamin D the body can't absorb calcium. Most of us get enough vitamin D from sunshine and milk, but if you are inside most of the time, wear heavy sun-screens when you're outside, and drink less than a quart of milk a day, it might be a good idea to take a multiple vitamin. This will give you 400 I.U. of vitamin D, which is the desired daily requirement.

Regular exercise also helps us absorb calcium. Eliza-beth says, "Activities such as brisk walking, treadmill, descending flights of stairs, dancing, or tennis are encour-aged. Clinical experience leads us to believe that three hours a week of this type of exercise can slow down the rate of bone loss, and activities like square dancing six hours a week can actually increase bone mass, even in the elderly.''

Elizabeth wraps up the consultation by telling me how important it is for young men and women in their twenties and early thirties "to make sure they do everything to achieve optimal bone mass.'' The bottom line is that the process that ends in bone loss and osteoporosis begins long before menopause and your first bone-density test. Women who eat right and get plenty of calcium and exercise in their earlier years build bone that is better able to withstand osteoporosis. It does not make me feel very good knowing that the best time for me to do something about osteoporosis was twenty years ago, especially since I didn't know better.

When I was in my twenties and thirties I never heard a word about this silent ladykiller. I never even knew there was such a thing as osteoporosis. When I saw a little old woman with a dowager's hump I just assumed you got shorter when you got older. What did I know about osteoporosis? I didn't read *Modern Maturity* or the *New England Journal of Medicine*. I read *Glamour* and *Cosmo*.

In my time the pages of *Glamour* and *Cosmo* were filled with articles about single women and multiple orgasms. The magazines told us what to do with split ends and bad relationships and lemons and avocados and vaginal odor. We read the poems of Rod McKuen, looked at the illustrations of Peter Max, and bought the promises of Mark Eden and his bust developer. They showed us how to make a fabulous fondue, wear a miniskirt, and look like Twiggy. They helped us get a man with guacamole, macramé, Cold Duck, and scones. They never said a word about calcium, exercise, and bones.

In my twenties thin was in. Women were encouraged to trade high-fat, calcium-rich dairy products for zero-calorie, calcium-robbing, phosphorus-filled diet soft drinks. No one told us it was dangerous. There weren't warning labels in all size-five dresses saying that the Surgeon-General warns that this size puts you at risk for osteoporosis. The magazines had us worrying about how we would look in a bathing suit when we should have been worrying about how we would look in a walker. The crime is we didn't know better.

This was a day that started with woulda, coulda, and shoulda, and ended much the same way. If I woulda' known about osteoporosis and calcium when I was younger I coulda' taken better care of my bones and I shoulda' known better than to think that all I had to do was pass the bone-density test and my problems would be over. That test didn't mark the end of my problems, but the beginning. This time I was 3 percent above normal but what about next time? There is a major hormonal shift taking place here and I am running low on estrogen. With estrogen it is not easy come, easy go. It is hard when it goes. My body misses it and my bones require it.

I have been trying to make menopause a natural, normal, positive experience but I am absolutely positive there is nothing natural or normal about porous bones and a shrinking skeleton.

When you are postmenopausal, diet and exercise are no substitute for estrogen in the prevention of bone loss. Clean living and a wholesome diet are no match for a deadly diabolical killer like osteoporosis. If diet and exercise met osteoporosis in a dark alley, you can be sure they would give him all your bone and beg for their lives. The only way I have a fighting chance is with estrogen. With diet and exercise my skeleton has an uncertain future. But if I bone up with estrogen it's definitely "sayonara osteoporosis." In this case an ounce of estrogen is worth a pound of prevention.

Both Elizabeth Treadwell and Dr. Brown, two professionals I respect, have great faith in the power of estrogen. According to them, HRT will take me from the hormonal hell of menopause and osteoporosis and deliver me to the carefree kingdom of hormonal heaven. All I have to do is swallow a couple of these divine little estrogen tablets and my hot flashes will disappear, my night sweats will dry up, my vagina will again be wet and moist, my bones won't turn to dust, and my heart won't attack me.

I know that I am being too dramatic, that I have blown this up to biblical proportions, that I am making too much of this. This is not a religious experience. This is a simple decision and I have made it into the Last Temptation of Gayle. But at this point I am not prepared to join the First Church of Estrogen. I'm afraid, for now, that I am a hormonal heretic.

SIX

Is It Hot in Here
or Is It Me?

I was not only a hormonal heretic, I was also a hormonal hermit. Menopause was supposed to be a natural, normal, liberating experience, yet it was turning me into a social shut-in. I no longer socialized for fear of the uncomfortable and embarrassing hot flash. The few times we went out for dinner it was to a restaurant that had great air-conditioning. We chose a restaurant not for the reviews but for the BTUs. Most of my free time I stayed home nursing my hot flashes and waiting for the pause to pass. Was I alone? Was I the only woman in North America held hostage by her hormones? To a woman in menopause the whole world is menopausal. I could not look at another woman without wondering if she was experiencing what I was. I even played an imaginary game where I tried to guess from her walk and her age and her attitude and her posture if she was having a hot flash or vaginal dryness or experiencing osteoporosis. I called the game What's My Menopause?

I watch MTV. Tina Turner sensually grinds out a song, the sweat pouring off her overheated body. Is it the music or a hot flash? Maybe both. I pick up a magazine and there is a picture of Jackie Kennedy on horseback. Would she be sitting on a horse if she had vaginal dryness? Maybe. She's a very courageous woman. Is Dr. Ruth short or is it osteoporosis? I don't know. I go to a casual restaurant where a short woman around fifty, in a full-length mink coat, is having a heated argument with her husband. Hot flash? Osteoporosis? Vaginal dryness? Ostentation? Probably all four.

The more I played the game the more I realized that I was not the only woman with a hot flash, a dry vagina, and a wet mattress. There were other women out there going through what I was going through and they were functioning. They were not letting their hormones push them around and affect the quality of their life. If Tina could sing and Jackie could ride and Ruth could counsel, then surely Gayle could party. So, when my menopause, my husband, and I were invited to a fancy dinner party I insisted that we all go. Life goes on even with hot flashes.

I would be going into this situation well aware of the consequences but I would be well prepared. I would give myself every chance of getting through the evening without succumbing to the dreaded hot flash. I would not allow myself to become terrorized by my hormones. The preparation was as meticulous and the planning as precise as my first wedding. There would be no slip-ups. Nothing would be overlooked. This was a formal dinner party so I could not wear a sweat suit. I would have to wear a dress. I chose a loose-fitting black summer cocktail dress. On the surface, I would be Donna Karan but underneath I will wear more layers than a bag lady. Makeup will be minimal and waterproof; hair simple and off the face; shoes will be sensible. I will also carry a designer bag containing a hair dryer, absorbent towels, and a fresh pair of cotton-crotch absorbent underwear.

At the party I will avoid anything that could possibly trigger a hot flash. I will stay away from smokers, avoid spicy foods, cocktails, wine, hot drinks, sweets, colas, cakes, and anything with sugar. What I do eat, I will eat slowly and near an open window if there is one. It is February in New York and hopefully the wind-chill factor will favor my condition. I will take every precaution. After that it is up to chance. Whatever happens, happens.

Whatever happens starts to happen about five minutes after I arrive at the party. The apartment is spacious and elegant but the room everyone congregates in is small, crowded, and stuffy. I don't have a prayer. As I am introduced to our host, the first wave strikes. I start to tingle as my spine, like some huge natural immersion heater, starts to boil my water and turn it into steam. I begin to glow as the hot salty water works its way out of my kettle and onto my skin. I try to remain cool and calm and casual as the water seeps through my cotton under-garments and starts flowing under my arms and over my back and across my forehead.

My genial host, unaware of the fall of my cotton Maginot Line, asks, "Would you like a cocktail? A glass of wine? What would you like?" What I would like is to take off all my clothes, open all the windows, and dive into a tub of ice. That's what I would like but I ask for "a little icewater, thank you." While our host gets me my drink I make my way to the bathroom. Once inside I throw open the window, stick my head out, and begin to suck in the cold, windy, arctic February air. As I do, my eyes start to tear, my nose starts to run, and I feel hot and cold at the same time like some human Baked Alaska. I try to assess the damage by looking at myself in the bath-room mirror, but it has steamed up. I towel off, loosen up, and am about to return to the open window when there is a knock on the door. I go to close the window. It won't close. The harder I try the hotter and wetter I get. I decide to deal with it by not dealing with it. If I wait maybe the knocking will stop. It doesn't. It gets harder and louder. I try again to close the window. It won't close. The bathroom is now colder than a meat locker. On the other side of the door angry sounds now accompany frantic knocks. I make one last try at closing the window.

It won't budge. I hastily clean up my mess and try to pull myself together without the aid of a mirror. I then open the door, apologize for the delay, and tell the person waiting about the open window. He is not interested. At this point he has more pressing problems. He quickly closes the door and I return to the party.

My nose is dripping, my eyes are tearing, but for now my flash is in remission. Waiting for me with a big glass of icewater is our host. I sip it daintily. I am once again the perfect guest. Our host then offers me some food. It is chili. I am taking no chances. I decline. He insists I try it. Wanting to remain the perfect guest I take a bite. The spicy food adds fuel to the flash and once again I glow and flow. As the water on the small of my back increases in circumference from a small a circle to the size of a beach ball I excuse myself and once again return to the comfort and warmth and security of the frigid bathroom. When I get there I am horrified. The window is closed. I don't dare open it again. I look in the mirror. It is not a pretty picture. I am a walking hot tub. My hair is glued to my scalp and looks like melted Jell-O, and there is a nice big wet patch on my stomach. I towel off, take out my hair dryer, turn on the tap water to muffle the sound, and make a lame attempt at drying my dress and my mess. As I try to pull myself together I'm thinking, What was I thinking when I thought I could get away with this?

For the remainder of the evening I pretend that nothing is happening when in fact everything is happening. Trying to hide a hot flash is like trying to hide an elephant. My lack of appetite, profuse sweating, and frequent trips to the bathroom do not go unnoticed. My host is aware of my problem, only I am sure he thinks my problem is drugs, not menopause, and that I need Betty Ford, not hormones.

As we drive home in a taxi with the windows wide open I cannot help but think what a complete fool I am. I do not take drugs. I do not even take hormones, and yet having our host think that I was an out-of-control drug addict was preferable to him thinking that I was having a natural, normal experience. This was not real life, this was sitcom. This was "Lucy Meets Menopause." I couldn't handle it anymore. I was not going to allow menopause and the hot flash to become the bonfires of my insanity. I was no longer going to pretend nothing was happening when everything was happening. No more denial. Time to go public.

The next morning I get on an elevator on my way to a dental appointment. As the car fills with passengers I start to perk, bubble, and drip. My first instinct is to get out immediately. I don't. To no one in particular, I ask, "Is it hot in here or is it me?" There are some nervous coughs, some people continue staring at the numbers, some look at me like I'm an extraterrestrial and get off at the next floor, some face forward making no eye contact, others pretend not to hear. There are also some real smiles of recognition from both men and women. I had broken the ice and it felt good. No guilt, no remorse, just relief.

When I tell my new dentist, Dr. Bruce Blau, that I am menopausal, he is very surprised. He picks, probes, sticks, shrugs, and says, "You couldn't tell from your mouth." When I tell him he's looking in the wrong place he laughs and tells me that my gums and vagina have the same tissue and that the loss of estrogen at menopause cannot only cause a dry vagina but also a dry mouth. I rinse. I nod. He continues. He tells me that another condition that can occur at menopause is Burning Mouth syndrome. Symptoms are a burning sensation in the tongue, floor of the mouth, hard palate, and cheeks. There is a decrease in the tolerance to heat and a bitter metallic taste. I nod, he aspirates, and then postulates. "You know, the first signs of osteoporosis are usually in the mouth. Many times you will lose bone in the jaw before the vertebrae." He continues looking in my mouth and I continue looking up his nose, and as he proceeds with his lecture on porous bones and dry vaginas he asks me questions that I cannot answer. The dentist's chair is the home of the rhetorical question. He tells me that he refers many of his postmenopausal patients not only to a periodontist but also to a gynecologist.

Postmenopausal women who are not on estrogen

therapy lose more bone and teeth than men. But those that are on HRT may get bleeding gums because increased levels of estrogen make gum tissue more vulnerable to plaque. Unless you really take good care of your teeth and gums you will get gingivitis and eventually periodontal disease. When we take a break from all the digging, sticking, probing, drooling, and rinsing, I tell him if he has any more unpleasant information to please give me a shot of Novocain first.

To be safe he suggests a set of full-mouth X rays. "It's a good idea, especially when you're menopausal and there's a chance of bone loss." When I tell him that I'm more concerned with radiation poisoning he tells me that the X rays are perfectly safe. He then proceeds to cover me with a lead bib, puts an X-ray film in my mouth, tells me to hold my breath, aims a nuclear warhead at my jaw, and races outside the room into what I presume is a lead bunker. I am ground zero. He is nowhere to be found. Sure X rays are safe, if you're not the patient. After repeating this process several times he once again looks deeply into my mouth and tells me I have beautiful pink and healthy gums. I might have a middle-aged vagina but at least I have young gums.

On the elevator down I do a gratuitous "Is it hot in here?" just to test my confidence. The two middle-aged couples in the elevator look at me like I just burned the flag.

Charlie, my fruit-and-vegetable man at Balducci's, is

a stocky Italian guy in his sixties. I've known Charlie most of my adult life. Every time he sees me he greets me the same way. "How's the best lookin' tomato in New York?" That's a very big compliment coming from a guy who really knows his produce. When I tell Charlie I'm going through menopause he congratulates me. "Hey, that's great! Now you're safe!"

"Charlie, stick to produce," I say.

He does. He tells me to buy some pomegranates and dates. They were used in biblical times in place of estrogen. Cleopatra ate them. "If it's good enough for the Queen of d'Nile it should be good enough for you, doll."

Later that day when I bring in my limp, sweat-stained black dress to the dry cleaners, Lillian, who runs the store with her husband, Murray, inspects it and asks me if I was in Florida. "Why Florida?" I ask. She explains that no one sweats like this in New York in February unless they're stuck in the subway during rush hour or somebody's chasing them. When I tell her I'm menopausal and this is the result of a hot flash, she nods sympathetically. Lillian is in her sixties and looks fantastic for her age. She wears loud prints and noisy jewelry. When she moves she rustles and jingles like a wind chime.

Lillian had instant menopause. A hysterectomy. "I already had six kids and I didn't want another. I was forty-four and my biggest fear was that I would have change-of-life quintuplets." She winks, smiles, and touches my arm to make her points. "When my gynecologist suggested we take out the baby carriage and leave the playpen it seemed like a good idea." He told her that she didn't need her uterus and without it she wouldn't have to worry about kids, menstrual cramps, periods, or uterine cancer.

At the time everybody was getting a hysterectomy. "They were as popular as mood rings and Hula Hoops. They were called 'Hollywood Appendectomies.' " Lillian was so sure she was doing the right thing she didn't even get a second opinion. It was supposed to be a simple hysterectomy—her uterus and cervix were to be removed but she was to keep her ovaries. Unfortunately, they found benign fibroid tumors on her ovaries and removed the ovaries along with the fibroids. After the operation she was sure her troubles would be over. They were just beginning. "I not only lost my uterus, I lost my mind."

All hell broke loose. "I was a bitch on wheels. I would have these wild mood swings. I'd go from weepy to crazy. One minute I'd be crying uncontrollably from something I saw on 'The Dating Game' and an hour later I'd get violent with someone who was standing in front of me on the express line in the supermarket with more than seven items. It was worse than labor. I would have preferred quintuplets. If not for estrogen therapy I wouldn't be here today."

Lillian tells me that not too long ago history was about to repeat itself. Her daughter Hillary, who is thirty-three, was having heavy menstrual bleeding and a sonogram revealed uterine fibroids. Her doctor recommended a hysterectomy despite her age and the fact that the fibroids were benign. It's been twenty years since Lillian's hysterectomy and apparently nothing's changed. Currently, there are 600,000 hysterectomies performed each year in this country. That's one every minute. That's sixty an hour. The national speed limit is fifty-five. In their rush to remove the uterus gynecologists are committing gynecide on our reproductive systems. The hysterectomy should be the final solution to the fibroid problem, not the first. The risks posed by surgery to remove fibroids are greater than those of the tumors themselves. Multiple uterine fibroids are as common as weeds but instead of cutting the grass the medical profession insists on chopping down the uterus and pruning the ovaries.

Hillary was still young, wanted to have children, and was not about to have a hysterectomy. She shopped around and found out she didn't have to. There are alternatives. She could have microsurgery or a myomectomy, which would remove the tumors and leave her reproductive system intact. Even with these options five out of six women who have surgery for fibroids have hysterectomies. Doctors say with the other procedures the fibroids can return. With the hysterectomy nothing returns, including your uterus and ovaries.

Some doctors will look for alternatives for young women like Hillary, but the medical profession has very little concern for the reproductive system of the older woman. If you are menopausal you'd better keep your eye on your uterus. If you don't you'll get it snatched faster than a purse on a New York street. Maybe I'm just a hopeless, sentimental romantic, but I'm in no hurry to part with my uterus. I'm hanging on for dear life. On the wall behind the counter of Lillian's store, neatly framed, is the first dollar she ever made. She kept it for luck. I plan to do the same with my uterus.

Diane liked menopause. It gave her the freedom to do what she wanted to do. "No more babies and no more little homemaker role for me." She had fulfilled her obligations and responsibilities as a wife and mother and now it was time to do what was good for Diane. It was time for a change. A real change. So Diane put in the wash, shopped, cleaned, dusted, straightened up, put everything away, turned out the lights and at forty-seven left her husband and twenty-five years of marriage for another woman. A menopausal woman. "It was great being with someone who actually could relate to what I was experiencing. It's nice when you and your mate are comfortable with the temperature." The only problem was that when one of them had a hot flash it caused a chain reaction. "Her flash would ignite mine and mine hers. We just kept igniting each other." Before they burned to a crisp, Diane and her menopausal mate split. She now

has a younger lover, there are no dueling hot flashes, and
things are much cooler. Now "good in bed" means not
soaking the sheets.

I met Diane when I visited her New Age book shop,
Dream Street. I spent many hours in her magical, sweet-
smelling, serene little shop talking about flatulence, bloat,
painful intercourse, and porous bones. Diane's mother
was only sixty-nine when she died from complications
from osteoporosis. "She had just retired and every time
she bent down to smell the roses she broke something."
That's why Diane started taking estrogen. Diane hates
pills, so she wears a transdermal patch on her stomach.
"It makes me look like a blow-up doll but it works." Her
period has returned and this pleases her: "It has mystical
significance, but mainly I had enough Tampax to last me
to the year 2014, and I really missed the mess." But she
missed little else from her past life. "I was tired of the
house, the car, the husband, and being the perfect pre-
heat-the-oven housewife." She took her job so seriously
she underlined the important parts of the cleanser instructions. "Even when we had sex I was his little love
slave—I had to get the candles and pour the wine and give
him a massage and change the sheets. Every time we
went to bed I set the woman's movement back a thousand years." Diane was a product of the "without a man
you're nothing" generation, but all that's changed. She
no longer needs a man and a marriage for security. "If I

want security I'll get a dog. I want something and someone more exciting and challenging and at my age there
are five great women for every mediocre man. I'd have to
be nuts to settle for some dull frog when there are so
many exceptional and available women around.''

Nora is a dark, beautiful, Type-A career super-
woman and she wasn't going to let her hormones be her
kryptonite. She would not allow herself to have menopause. She was not about to lose her youth, her career,
and her boyfriend. Nora is on HRT. ''It's tough enough
being a woman in business,'' she says. ''Being a menopausal woman is too much of a liability.'' A woman in
business must not only be able to produce, she must be
able to reproduce. ''If my associates knew I was too old
to have children they would look at me differently. If I
can't use my sexuality I will lose power and will wind up
being one of those industrial housewives who make coffee and order lunch.'' They want bright young, not dull
old.

''With all due respect to the woman's movement, it's
dog eat dog out there or should I say puppy eats dog.
Youth is everything and in the business world a hot flash
doesn't exactly win friends and influence people.'' Nora
was in no position to educate her peers in the fundamen-
tals of vasomotor disturbances. ''They will use it against
me as proof that I can't function.'' Until attitudes in the
workplace change, dressing for success includes estro-

gen. "Sometimes I get so depressed and frustrated that I want to kill myself. The only thing that stops me is that they would print my age in the obituary. I couldn't live with that." I did not need a memo to get Nora's message.

Ramona, my menopausal manicurist, doesn't believe in nature. She believes in "plastic." She doesn't take vacations; she makes trips to doctors to get "things done." She's had a little nip, a little tuck, and a lot of silicone. She has had her face lifted with surgery and her spirits lifted with estrogen. "The stuff makes me feel good. I love those little oval-shaped burgundy beauties. They are the one pill I never forget to take." Ramona does not believe in exercise. Instead of going from the menstrual cycle to the exercycle she went to liquid diets, fat magnets, and liposuction. She is convinced that riding an escalator without holding on is aerobic. Ramona is an expert on the unnatural. She knows everything about tightening, loosening, lengthening, pointing, blunting, nipping, and tucking. She believes in the quick fix and microwave medicine. Between appointments, she studies the pictures of the celebrities in magazines like *People* and *Vanity Fair* and makes comments like "Great nose," "Nice tuck," "Lousy lift." Ramona even has cosmetic guidelines. "With a good lift you look well-rested. A bad lift looks like you should rest in peace." With Ramona, plastic surgery is a blood sport.

Between doing my nails, sipping on Diet Cokes, and

sneaking cigarettes in the back of the salon she tells me that I am crazy not to take hormones for my menopause. "Don't be a martyr. Take as much estrogen as is legal and then take more. Why go with nature when you've got cosmetics, surgery, hormones, and chemicals at your disposal." When I tell her my disposal is what I'm afraid of and that I think HRT is risky she tells me that everything is risky: "Honey, I just read where eating a handful of potato chips every day can take seven months off your life and smoking a pack of cigarettes a day is safer than a divorce. I bet riding a New York subway has got to be more dangerous than a lifetime supply of estrogen." After weighing all the facts Ramona decided to stay away from potato chips, not get a divorce, never take the IRT, BMT, and IND, but to take HRT.

The more I talked about it, the more everyone talked about it. It felt great not having a secret anymore. Besides, there was nothing to hide. Menopause is a fact of life. I got so secure with it that I even had the audacity to go to the main branch of the New York Public Library, approach a young male librarian, and whisper at the top of my lungs, "Where's the menopause section?" I then brazenly hung around 618.1, which in case you didn't know is Dewey Decimal for menopause, and even checked out a few of the books. Later, in broad daylight on an uptown bus, I recklessly took out the books and shamelessly flipped through them in full view of total strangers. I had come a long way from that first flash in L.A.

It was easy being a menopausal woman in New York because New York is a menopausal city. It is hot and cold and wet and it never sleeps. It is used to growth and change and atrophy and decay and anxiety. In New York middle age doesn't creep up on you. It confronts you every day, smacks you in the face and makes you deal with it.

After all was said and done I realized that going around the city flashing my menopause like some hormonal pervert wasn't really dealing with it. Going public with my privates wasn't enough. Shouting "Hey, look at me, I'm over the hill!" wasn't exactly coming to grips with menopause and middle age. Dealing with it meant getting off the menopausal merry-go-round and facing the facts.

The facts are that I am forty years older than my house, forty-eight years older than my car, and the same age as the movie *Casablanca*. I am considerably younger than the Statue of Liberty but I will never be Miss Teenage U.S.A., Mother of the Year, or a Supreme Court Justice. The fact is I won't even be a Supreme. Right now I am sitting in the middle of what my life turned out to be. According to statistics I have thirty years ahead of me without the protection of estrogen and without it anything can happen. Will I change? Get wrinkles? Lose my gums and teeth? Dry up? Get a divorce? Give birth with a donated egg? Start wearing sensible shoes and selling Amway? Who knows? What I do know is that it's time to get real. Get a life. Make some choices.

Ramona, Diane, Nora, and Lillian all made choices. They all chose to keep the hormones coming and to make the change no change. All had good reasons and HRT worked for them. Now it's my turn to decide. Do I want to push nature out of the way with man-made chemicals? Do I want to join the Hormone Protection Program and get new hormones, a new life, and a new start? I have come out of the closet but I am definitely not out of the woods.

SEVEN

New Age for Middle Age

My name is Gayle X and I'm a junkie. An estrogen junkie. I've been on the stuff all my life. My body needs it. I can't function without it. It calms me down. It makes me feel good. It gives me sexual power. It makes me feel like a woman. When I was on it I was on top of the world. I had it all—youth, fresh skin, a sex life, a period. But all that's changed. My supply has dried up. My source has gone out of business. My ovaries have been busted. Nature's drug supply has been cut off. I'm having withdrawal symptoms . . . hot flashes, cold sweats, insomnia, anxiety, the shakes. All the classic signs of withdrawal. As I lie in bed soaking wet, wearing my damp sheets like pedal pushers, I realize I have hit bottom. Hormonal Hell. Until now I didn't realize how strung out I was on estrogen. How much my body needed it just to function normally. How important it was to me. I must kick this estrogen dependency and move on.

All my life I've been under the influence of estrogen. Maybe it's time to look at life without it. Right now I don't want any drugs or quick fixes. There has got to be an alternative to HRT. Surely, if God in all his wisdom wanted us to replace our lost estrogen he wouldn't have hidden it in the urine of a horse. There has got to be another way to face the future. It's time to dry out and find out.

I begin my twelve-step program by going through my closets and drawers and gathering my estrogen para-phernalia. I throw out my Tampax and flush my Midol and birth control down the toilet. It's hard to throw away this link with my addiction but I can't keep it around and it's not exactly the stuff you give to Goodwill Industries. When you are coming off estrogen it is not a time to be emotionally isolated. It's important to share your deepest secrets with other women. It is six in the morning. Too early to bond but I must keep moving. I get dressed and go to the gym.

Dottie has the locker next to mine. I thought I knew everything about this naked woman next to me but I really knew nothing. She was menopausal-age but we never discussed it. I would never ask another woman about her menopause because it implies that she looks menopausal. Women find this very insulting because they all think they look twenty-two, including me. But on this morning I was desperate. I had to talk. When I talked she opened right up. A few months ago, Dottie had been having hot flashes every hour on the hour. She was like Old Faithful. The women in her office would look at her and know what time it was. "It's three hot flashes to lunch." She also felt bloated and was very irritable because the night sweats kept her from sleeping. When she told her doctor, he wanted to put her on estrogen immediately. She had been taking the Pill all her life and didn't want to take any more hormones. Instead, she went to an acupuncturist to relieve her symptoms.

I always thought of acupuncture as just a painkiller, the Chinese answer to Novocain. Dottie tells me that they use it to treat everything from drug addiction to hot flashes. Medically, acupuncture has more uses than a Cuisinart. Dottie went for a couple of months and took the needles and tried the different herbs. "I started out with dong quai, which is the female ginseng, but it is very potent stuff and made me irritable. So I tried black cohosh but that didn't work either." What finally did work was a sage tea made with sage, blue vervain, motherwort, blessed thistle, rosemary, and ginseng. She drank several cups a day and it did the trick.

Dottie tells me she no longer has hot flashes and night sweats and is sleeping soundly. She looks great and she isn't moody and cranky at work. The only problem is that now the women in the office don't know when to go to lunch. I am ambivalent about Dottie's approach to menopause. Ginseng may be natural but it is still estrogen and it has the same effect on your body as taking the hormones her doctor prescribed. Unfortunately, with ginseng, you can't tell how much estrogen you are getting, so it's possible to O.D. Also, you don't get the protection of progesterone that you get with HRT. I know ginseng is natural but that doesn't mean it's safe. Many people die of natural causes.

It's only been a couple of months since Dottie found her cure, but who knows? Maybe the symptoms will return and because it works for Dottie doesn't mean it will work for me. I'm always reading stories about men who are cured of cancer by watching Three Stooges movies and others who keep tropical fish because it lowers their high blood pressure. You never read about how many of these movie watchers died laughing or how many aquarium starers are now dead as a mackerel. Maybe none. But for now I'm keeping my options open.

Ruth, a spunky little fifty-year-old blonde, also belonged to the gym, and after our workouts we started comparing notes on our latest menopausal symptoms. Our daily exchanges helped us to put things in perspective. We would always ask each other, "Is it real or is it menopause? Is this me talking or is it my out-of-control hormones?" We both knew that this was not a time to be emotionally isolated, that it was important to share our deepest secrets, to bond. The men had Robert Bly, we had each other. It was great to let our thinning, graying hair down and not be judged or laughed at. Neither of us was on HRT so the only relief we got was from empathy and sympathy.

Ruth took her sore breasts, hot flashes, bloating, and snoring in stride. She even made jokes about her incontinence. When her gynecologist suggested kegels—vaginal toning exercises—for bladder control, Ruth had a problem. "He told me to contract my sphincter muscle. Contract it? I can't even contact it. For the last week, I've tried getting in touch with it every hour of the day but it's never home." There was one thing that Ruth did not find funny and that was her dry vagina and the itching and especially the odor that came with it. She tried everything—feminine hygiene spray, every genital deodorant: Norforms, Feminique, Eve, FDS Towelettes. She even tried Listerine and Head and Shoulders. I suggested she stop trying to hide it, mask it, and spray it. To get to the source, see a doctor.

She didn't see a doctor but she did see an herbologist, who gave her a vaginal gel made out of the herb slippery elm, which she inserted once a day. She also took a tincture of chickweed—thirty drops several times a day. She did this for three weeks and the odor disappeared. To help prevent yeast infections she ate and applied yogurt and inserted acidophilus capsules five hours before making love. The acidophilus is great for lubrication but the best thing for a dry vagina is sex. Her herbologist told her,

"It's kegeling with a partner." Fortunately her partner was easier to find than her sphincter.

Joan is an instructor at the gym where I met Ruth and Dottie. She is in her sixties, with very short cropped hair, well built, dangerous looking. To look at her you'd think career military, retired. She could also be right at home on a motorcycle, hanging on to some bearded, black-leather wild man as they race to get his-and-hers tattoos. One day, Joan happened to be changing next to Ruth and me as we were discussing Ruth's problems. When she heard what we were talking about she opened right up. She was very proud of Ruth for airing her problems. "When I was going through menopause nobody had the guts to talk about it. We used to call menopause the silent service." It turns out that Joan is not tough and hard. She is warm and caring. She is sixty-seven, has six kids, has never been in the army, drives a Datsun station wagon, doesn't have a single tattoo, and teaches yoga.

She learned her yoga not in New Delhi but in New Jersey, and though she appeared to look more at home on a Harley than in an ashram she was a true believer. She came to yoga by way of menopause. "My children were driving me nuts, my husband was driving me nuts, my menopause was driving me nuts." She was outnumbered. She just couldn't sleep or relax. When HRT didn't work she tried everything else—Midol, Nytol, Tylenol, Nyquil, Elavil, and Tofranil. Before she got to Valium,

Librium, and a sanitarium she went to a gymnasium, started taking yoga lessons, and never stopped.

Joan now teaches Hatha Yoga, which is physical yoga. She told me that there were specific exercises for menopause and that in three months I would be a new person. "If you come for lunch you'll stay for life."

I had heard about yoga from friends and I had read about it in magazines. Yoga is the oldest existing physical culture system in the world. It was here 5,000 years before Jane, Jake, Jack, videos, and free introductory offers but it always seemed a little too mystical for me. Whenever someone mentioned yoga I always thought of some Gandhi-like swami serenely lying on a bed of nails or casually walking through a bed of white-hot coals. I was never really interested in mastering either of these disciplines. But times have changed and right now I am going through the changes. If it can help an Indian fakir get through hot coals, maybe it can help me get through my hot flashes. If I can learn to sit on a bed of nails, then painful sex ought to be a piece of cake.

Joan's "ashram" is a little room tucked in the back of the gym. When I get there the students are milling around waiting for Joan, the guru. The group is decidedly nonspiritual. It looks more like jury duty than a yoga class. There is a forty-year-old tough truck-driver type wearing a black T-shirt sawed off above his bulging biceps. A couple of middle-aged housewives, a receptionist, an accountant, a young actor, and two peppy old gray-haired men who appeared to be very fond of each other. The students are friendly and warm but the room is very hot. It isn't me. Yoga studios are warm to keep your muscles pliable. When Joan arrives we each take a mat and remove our shoes. In yoga you don't wear shoes. This is a first—a land-based activity that Nike or Reebok doesn't make a shoe for. After we are all settled on our mats Joan dims the lights and plays some New Age Zen water music by some all-crystal sitar quintet and we begin.

I should say, they begin. As Joan leads the class in the first position I become instantly aware of my body's limitations. I try to do the posture. I want to do the posture but my mind is not communicating with my muscles. They are not responding to the messages from my brain. There is no connection; the lines are dead. What's worse, at this point I don't even know what part of my body to contact that would put me in touch with these muscles. I feel like I am stuck inside my body, all alone, out of gas, in the middle of nowhere. I am thinking to myself that this exercise is impossible and incomprehensible; nobody can do this. When I look around I see that everybody is doing it. I am flopping and floundering and swaying while they are slipping effortlessly in and out of the positions. Frustrated, my brain frantically presses the keys on my muscular keyboard. But I am not getting music. All I am getting is noise. Everyone encourages me. But all the attention makes me self-conscious and it gets worse. It is hopeless. I thought yoga was designed to reduce stress, not cause it. The pursuit of tranquillity and serenity can be a frightening experience.

After the class I tell Joan how disappointed I am. I have been exercising all my life and thought that yoga was going to be a breeze. I expected my body to bend like a paper clip, not just sit there like a paperweight. Joan tells me not to be discouraged, that the students with the most trouble get the most out of it, because they have to concentrate more and work harder. "Don't be impatient. Whatever you do, you'll do better tomorrow. It's the effort, not the performance, that counts. Keep coming and I will teach you how to breathe and how to do the pump, the spinal flex, the wide-angle pose, the plow, the upward-facing dog, and the locust." These are the postures that are great for all the menopausal symptoms. The locust not only energizes the entire female reproductive system; it is also great for varicose veins and hemorrhoids. I tell her I will return to learn the locust, yoga's answer to Preparation H.

There are supposed to be 840,000 yoga exercises. In the next two weeks I learn thirty-three. Yoga is helping me to sleep better and be more relaxed but I haven't gotten to the walk-on-a-bed-of-white-hot-coals stage yet. Right now I am still having trouble with the walk-on-a-

bathroom-floor-of-ice-cold-tiles phase of my yogic progress. I believe I am something like 839,967 positions
away from that achievement. But until that milestone is
reached life goes on. I cook, clean, go to work, attend
more yoga classes, but continue to flash and sweat.

One frigid February morning I bring my car in for
service. While waiting to talk to a mechanic I have a hot
flash. As I stand there in that unheated garage, beet-red,
face flushed, fanning myself with my warranty book,
standing opposite me is a woman, beet-red, face flushed,
fanning herself with her warranty book. Instant recognition. Instant connection. Instant friends. I'll never forget
it. Millie doesn't remember it, but then Millie doesn't
remember a lot of things.

My friend Millie is a first-class travel agent whose
memory took a vacation during menopause. She could
remember the license plate numbers of every one of her
boyfriends' cars, what she had for breakfast every day of
her honeymoon, the lyrics to every single Connie Francis
song, but she couldn't remember to confirm a reservation
or return a phone call. She would write notes to herself
and the next day forget what they meant. "I wrote this?
Can't be." It got so bad that on some days she even forgot
how to use her computer. In the travel business your
computer is your life. You use it to locate accommoda-
tions and make reservations. "I'd sit in front of that keyboard trying to book someone into the San Juan Hilton

and I'd be paralyzed. I'm asking my brain to get me into the computer and all I'm getting back is the lyrics to an old Connie Francis tune. The client is screaming for dates and rates and all my brain is able to come up with is, 'Who's sorry now? Who's heart is aching for breaking each vow?' I'm losing customers and all I hear is 'Who's sad and blue? Who's crying, too?' The harder I try the worse it gets. I ask my brain to tell me what keys to punch for a room rate and all I can come up with is, 'You had your way. Now you must pay. I'm glad that you're sorry now.' I am no longer a travel agent. I am a juke box.''

After a day of trying to remember everything she forgot, Millie would go home and relax with her hot flashes, night sweats, heart palpitations, anxiety attacks, and insomnia. She was a wreck. ''My brain was fuzzy all the time.'' If this continued she would lose her job. She was under a lot of pressure and the harder she tried the worse it got. She tried mnemonic devices, notes, tapes, riddles, rhymes, even string. Nothing worked. Millie wanted to take estrogen. Her doctor advised her against it because she had gall bladder disease.

She was completely stressed out. In desperation she bought a Syncro Energizer. It's a device that uses light and sound to make you relax. You lie on your back, put the goggles over your eyes and listen to New Age music over the headphones while lights inside the goggles flash on and off, sending out waves of warmth and relaxation.

I tried it. It's like being in a meditation disco. This is not Nirvana. This is Nintendo. When I told Millie to try yoga she wasn't interested. She was caught up in the electronics and gadgetry. She tried flotation tanks, isolation chambers, and finally settled on biofeedback. By hooking up to a machine she was able to control her alpha waves and reduce stress. This also helped cool her hot flashes. Basically, it's yoga with electrodes, but it worked. Millie started relaxing more, sleeping sounder, and with brain foods like Ginkgold and lecithin she started functioning again. For her other menopausal symptoms her chiropractor recommended 800 I.U. of vitamin E with selenium and bioflavonoids in combination with vitamin C. Bioflavonoids have the same chemical structure as estrogen but are one-fifty-thousandth the strength. For fatigue and emotional swings she took a 200 mg tablet of potassium and magnesium aspartate. For her dry vagina she would break open a vitamin E capsule and apply the contents directly to her vagina. Things have gotten so good for Millie that now she can't remember that she couldn't remember.

Fortunately, my brain hadn't turned to Teflon but I must admit that I was helped considerably by daily reminders that I used to ignore or resent. I was now grateful for the "Have you enclosed your check?" reminders that came with the electric bill, and the "Have you forgotten anything?" sign posted in the taxicab and the "Fasten seat belt" and "You left your key in the ignition" and "Lights on" warnings in my car. I was even thankful for the sixty-three "Have you forgotten to renew your subscription?" notices from a magazine I don't remember ever subscribing to.

Millie had her memory back and her biofeedback and her bioflavonoids but I had my yoga. It calmed me down, made me relax, sucked the stress right out of me. It made me feel good. I figured if once a week made me feel good then twice a week could make me feel twice as good. In a month I went from once to twice to five times a week. I couldn't get enough. I even did it at home. Whenever I got the urge I would sneak off somewhere, take off my shoes, open my mat, and do the locust or the plow or the pump or whatever would turn me on. I needed it. I couldn't live without it. I had a new addiction. I was hooked on yoga.

I was not alone. There were others who came to yoga class every day. There was one woman in the class who performed the most intricate exercises effortlessly and flawlessly. She did all the advanced postures as well as any double-jointed Indian swami. She moved slowly and easily and confidently. She was incredibly flexible, beautifully built and I figured she was either a professional dancer or had a genetic predisposition to twist herself into a pretzel. When I asked her how she got to yoga I was expecting to hear the word "maharishi." Instead, I heard the word "menopause." Sharon looked twenty but was forty and had hit menopause at thirty-eight. The average age for menopause is fifty-one. Forty-five is considered early. Thirty-eight is ridiculous. Her mother stopped menstruating at thirty-five. She tells me it was part heredity but mostly stress. "I was a mess. I had just gone through a bitter divorce and I now had to support three teenagers, one dog, two cats, three hamsters, a ten-room house, a thirty-year mortgage, and a twelve-year-old station wagon."

Sharon smoked, drank, was overweight, depressed, and bitter. "My ex-husband was out dating teenagers and I was home cleaning lint filters. I was thirty-eight and already a menopause poster girl. I spent all my time throwing open windows and ripping off my clothes. I planned my day around my hot flashes and my refrigerator. I was told that full-bodied women had much less trouble with menopause." Instead of taking hormones Sharon took rum raisin ice cream and raised her chances for breast cancer and a heart attack.

Sharon's gynecologist advised against hormones because she was thirty pounds overweight, had high blood pressure, and her mother had breast cancer. But because of her premature menopause she was at greater risk for osteoporosis, heart attack, and stroke if she didn't take hormones. Instead of taking a leap off a bridge, Sharon saw a naturopath. She had had success with one years before in treating her PMS. Naturopathic doctors believe in natural health and nutritional supplements. They emphasize life-style changes over drug therapy and surgery. Naturopaths train for four years like M.D.s but they are N.D.s, and can't write prescriptions.

Sharon's naturopath took all the conventional medical tests—Pap smear, breast exam, lipid counts, and bone-density test. He also told her she was an apple. Maybe you can't compare apples and oranges but you can definitely compare apples and pears. Apple-shaped women carry their excess weight around the waist and upper body and have greater risk for breast cancer, high blood pressure, diabetes, premature heart attack, and strokes than pear-shaped women, who pack their adipose on thighs and hips. To keep the doctor away Sharon, the Apple, would have to stop smoking, drinking, lose thirty pounds, go on a vegetarian diet, get plenty of exercise, and reduce stress.

Because Sharon was so young and already menopausal he recommended Pro-Gest, a natural treatment for her menopausal symptoms and osteoporosis. Pro-Gest is a topically applied natural progesterone that is dissolved in a moisturizing cream. It bypasses the liver and there are no toxic effects. The source of the natural progesterone is the barbasco plant, a giant wild yam found in Mexico. The cream has been used in Europe for many years. The doctors here think it's too weak but her doctor had great success with it and assured her that when given in adequate doses it is just as effective as synthetic hormones without the undesirable side effects.

Sharon's naturopath also told her that the best natural defense against osteoporosis is to keep the acidity of the blood in proper balance. If you don't, your body will be removing calcium from your bones to keep the pH balance in the blood. We all worry about the pH balance in our shampoo. Blood acidity isn't caused by bad shampoo. It is caused by chronic stress. Any woman over forty-five with high stress should stop smoking, drinking alcohol, coffee, and sodas, and start practicing yoga or another antistress technique.

Sharon chose yoga and it changed her life. "It got me out of myself and out of the house." In three months Sharon went from Den Mother to Zen Mother. Her diet went from micro to macro and she went from broom to Om. She gets a bone-density test every year and so far she's doing fine, not only medically but domestically. Her kids now clean their own rooms, butter their own toast, and match their own socks. Sharon not only taught her children how to operate all the appliances, she also taught them yoga. Whenever I visited her home it was nice to see the family lined up standing on their heads, eating brown rice, or meditating.

I visit Sharon often. She helps me with the headstand and the more advanced postures. She is my guru.

Because of her increased risk of osteoporosis and need for calcium I casually ask her how much milk she drinks. To which Sharon casually replies, "I don't drink milk, I don't believe in it." When she suggests I stop drinking it I don't know how to respond. As far as I'm concerned it's downright un-American to bad-mouth milk. I am tempted to defend cow and country from this milk bashing, bovine Benedict Arnold but maybe this is some kind of Eastern religious thing. This is all new to me. Up until now the only Oriental philosophy I've been exposed to was in fortune cookies. I simply ask, "What's wrong with milk?"

Sharon curdles, "Nothing—if you're a cow. But everything if you're a human. Our bodies weren't meant to drink cow's milk. No other species gets its milk from cows. They nurse their young with their own milk and we should do the same." I concede that maybe breast is best but that it is not exactly practical or legal or moral for someone my age to be getting their calcium from a human breast. She agrees but adds that I would be wise to find another source because there's an excellent chance that as I get older I will lose the ability to digest milk. According to Sharon most of the people in the world cannot properly digest milk. They are either allergic to it or intolerant to the lactose (milk sugar) in it. In some parts of the world it is even considered unfit for human consumption. If this is true I am in deep trouble.

Milk has become an important part of my life. My corn flakes float in it, my calcium swims in it, and I'm sunk without it.

Sharon says cows don't have a monopoly on calcium. In most of the world dairy products are not part of the diet. In Central America they mix lime with cornmeal to make calcium-rich tortillas. Tofu, a staple of Japanese cuisine, is rich in calcium. The average daily intake of calcium in all these no-dairy societies can easily reach 1,200–2,000 mg a day.

She takes out a clear plastic bag, digs her hand in, and gives me a handful of soft burgundy leaves, called dulce. It is seaweed. I put some in my mouth and start chewing. The taste is definitely briny, but pleasant. Sharon tells me that it is loaded with calcium, protein, iron, chlorophyll enzymes, and a lot more fiber than oat bran. It's not bad but it is no replacement for milk. It will do nothing for my corn flakes and it definitely won't wash down a handful of Oreos. For certain things there is just no substitute for a nice cold glass of high-calorie, fat-filled, cholesterol-heavy, lactose-laden cow's milk.

When I tell Sharon that I don't want to chew seaweed for the rest of my natural life, she suggests that I see Michael Abhaile at the health food store. I am a little skeptical. The health food store is not exactly the Mayo Clinic. I have difficulty taking nutritional advice from a doctor who only gets about twenty hours of nutritional education in medical school. But that's still twenty hours more than some eighteen-year-old kid who is working part-time in a health food store so that he can earn enough money to go to beauty parlor college at night. I take my vitamins and herbs very seriously. And I'm not about to put my life in the hands of someone who works in a business that is about as carefully regulated as the savings and loan industry. Sharon reassures me. "He's had formal training in macrobiotics and herbs and you'll be surprised at what he can come up with." When I tell her that maybe I'm a milkaholic and can't get off the stuff she insists that I go. "I promise you, you won't be sorry."

The next day I visited the health food store to meet Michael Abhaile. Inside it is cool and clean and small. There are a few display racks filled with natural organic foods, healthy snacks, and New Age doodads. But the main attraction here is not the display racks but the lunch counter. It is clear pine, heavily lacquered, and fills most of the store. This lunch counter even has its own name. A large dark green sign on the light green wall behind the counter reads THE JADED PALATE. Working behind the counter is Michael. He is tall and thin and young and in his crisp, fresh, white uniform and chef's hat he looks anything but jaded.

Milk is not a sacred cow to Michael either. He tells me he wouldn't touch the stuff. "It's the world's most overrated nutrient." Michael believes that you can get all the bone-building calcium you need from vegetables and seaweed. He shows me some seaweed and tells me that in one-quarter pound of raw seaweed like wakame there are 1,300 mg of calcium and as much as 1,400 in hijiki. "I don't know exactly how much is absorbed but there is so much that even a little will give you a lot of calcium."

"That's great but how do you eat this stuff?" I ask.

"Let me show you," he says.

As he prepares the seaweed I am shocked at his equipment. All he has is a hot plate. He cooks everything on a simple little primitive two-burner hot plate. As he mixes, stirs, chops, cuts, peels, and dices he moves pots and pans on and off the hot plate with the precision and rhythm and showmanship of one of those Hungarian plate-spinning acts that used to be on the "Ed Sullivan Show." He has it all worked out. He is a study in time and motion. Michael is a real chef. This isn't some kid in brown polyester with a funny hat who slaps your order together and makes change. This is not mass-produced, franchised, off-the-rack cooking. This is handmade food and it was made to order for my jaded palate. Michael has turned the humble hot plate into a haute plate.

In a matter of minutes he prepares a delicious-looking stir-fried teriyaki tempeh with ginger, mushrooms, scallions, and toasted sesame oil. With it he serves his special Better Bones and Garden Salad that has brown rice, arame, carrots, cauliflower, broccoli, squash, tamari, and tons of toasted sesame and pumpkin seeds. He presents it all with great style and when he places it in front of me says, "Bone appétit." It is "to die" health food. Michael mixes information in with the cooking. He tells me there is enough calcium in just the arame and the tempeh to give me 1,000 mg of calcium. He also tells me that the sesame seeds are loaded with calcium but in order to release the calcium you have to grind the seeds or roast them. As Michael shares his secrets I constantly interrupt with obscene little sighs and moans each time I bite into something new and wonderful. This is without a doubt the healthiest, best-tasting food I ever had. This isn't just great cooking. This is Cordon Bleu Cross Cooking.

Michael promises me that next time he will make his Hijiki Yam Ball Bone-Builders that have 1,400 mg of calcium. If I have a sweet tooth he will make me his Bone, Sweet Bone Lemon Apricot Kanten that has apples and raisins and is loaded with calcium. Kanten, also known as agar-agar, is the sea's answer to gelatin. Having total faith in this plate healer, I ask him what he has for menopause. Without saying a word he turns on a fan, points it at me, and proceeds to make me an iced herb tea. "I call this my Hot Flash Fizz," he says. It's made with Siberian ginseng, fennel, red raspberry, blessed thistle, black cohosh, wild yam root, and anise. It is delicious. Some of these herbs are said to have natural estrogen. When I ask him how he knows so much about menopause he tells me very matter of factly that his girlfriend is going through it. Before I choke on my fizz he winks and smiles and says, "Her mother is going through it." As his natural organic faithful followers begin filtering in for lunch I know it is time to leave The Jaded Palate. Michael and his heavenly hot plate have other palates to please.*

I am not certain that the Hot Flash Fizz can replace estrogen and that seaweed is a substitute for milk or that yoga will even take away my night sweats. I do know that the fizz is refreshing, seaweed tastes briny, and yoga makes me feel great. With it my body produces natural opiates and I'm much more relaxed. But this is not enough. I need more than the rush of endorphins. I need something stronger. I need something less mainstream and more mainline. I need something that packs a bigger wallop than yoga. Something that will be faster-acting and give more instant relief. I attend yoga classes five times a week, yet I still have all my menopausal symptoms. I have mastered all the menopause postures including the difficult headstand but according to my latest figures I am 839,808 exercises short of being able to walk through menopause. It is time to experiment with other natural alternatives.

I know that very little research has been done on the

*See Notes for Michael Abhaile's Cordon Bleu Cross Bone-Building Recipes.

alternatives to HRT and that most of the success stories are only stories and don't meet the random double-blind studies that are the bedrock of scientific medicine, but I would have to be completely blind and have rocks in my head if I ignored the success Millie, Joan, Sharon, Dottie, and Ruth had with their alternative experiences.

These women aren't desperate, hopeless flakes. This is not the I-was-kidnapped-by-Martian-endodontists-and-given-root-canal crowd. These are intelligent, reasonable, clear-thinking, hardworking, responsible, practical women with 2.6 children and 1.5 cars. These women don't believe in voodoo economics or waste money on snake oils that health insurance doesn't pay for. They aren't impressed by hucksters that bend spoons or witch doctors and chicken sacrifices. They don't wear copper bracelets, read tea leaves, attend seances, own Ouija boards or tarot cards, or call 900-number astrologers and psychics. These women are not alone. The fact is that 80 percent of menopausal women don't take hormones. Some can't take them for medical reasons; others won't take them for personal reasons. Conventional medicine is just another alternative. It is not the only choice.

Some of the alternatives aren't 100-percent safe, but neither is estrogen. None have been studied under the scrutiny of the double blind but many have passed the test of time. Acupuncture has been around 4,500 years, yoga

5,000. The world had been using herbs thousands of years before our doctors developed waiting rooms and invented malpractice insurance. After you stand on your head, you realize there is more than one way to stop a hot flash.

EIGHT

They Got the Whole Gayle in Their Hands

My husband and I bought a little vacation home in St. Augustine, Florida, the oldest city in the United States. It is over four hundred years old but it definitely isn't menopausal. In the last year I have had more changes than St. Augustine has had since it was founded by the Spanish in 1565.

I was living on the beach, avoiding milk and sipping Hot Flash Fizzes, but the change of life-style had very little effect on my change of life. I still had a dry vagina and the hot flashes rolled in every day with the consistency and energy of the tides. The only difference was that now they had an ocean view. I was discouraged but I wasn't giving up. I was still determined to find an alternative to estrogen.

When I told my husband that I was thinking about a nonmedical, more spiritual, holistic approach to my menopause, he was less than supportive: "You don't believe in that New Age stuff, do you?" The way he said it you'd think I was talking about leprechauns and tooth fairies. Medically my husband is more conservative than the AMA. He believes that if you are not an M.D. you are a fraud, a charlatan, a shaman, and a direct descendant of Rasputin. "Why don't you go to a real doctor, not some guy who got his degree from a school that advertises on matchbook covers?" When I remind him that holistic medicine has been around a lot longer than doctors and golf, he is not impressed.

"If I'm sick I don't want some recent graduate of the Cincinnati School of Truck Driving and Magnetic Healing playing with my chakras. If I've got pneumonia I'm going to the drugstore, not the health food store, and I'm swallowing large doses of penicillin, not herb tea. When you are sick you want medication, not meditation."

I agree, but I am not *sick*. I don't have an illness or a disease. To a doctor I am an estrogen-starved woman with failed ovaries and a senile atrophied vagina. Nature is not the enemy here. I don't need a doctor. All I want to do is see someone who will treat me like a normal healthy menopausal woman.

He still doesn't get it: "Don't you think it takes a tremendous leap of faith to believe that some guy who went to school for a weekend and tells you to take two crystals and call him in the morning can actually help you?'' He is way out of line. You need a lot more faith when you see a doctor. I tell him that only a medical Moonie would let a total stranger, in a mask, put him to sleep, cut him open, take something out, sew him back up, and charge him more money than he can afford. Menopause is not something that I have to fight, kill, or wipe out. I don't need armed intervention, I need passive resistance.

My hairdresser, Sylvie, a very spiritual vegetarian, suggested that I visit Hilda, a spiritual healer. According to Sylvie, Hilda is the real thing: ''She was struck by lightning when she was three, was meditating at four, and was healing pets at five. They even wrote her up in the *National Enquirer.*'' The *Enquirer* is not exactly the *New England Journal of Medicine* but I was still impressed. I think you should get a second opinion, even with faith healers, so I asked around. I spoke to several of the healer's satisfied healees and they all said the same thing: ''Let Hilda lay hands on your menopause.''

My husband does not believe in mind over matter. ''If I want to stop a car I'll take brakes over thoughts any day,'' he muttered. According to him, it just doesn't make sense. According to me, it doesn't have to. It is time for a little spiritual intervention.

Hilda lives in a little weatherbeaten house on stilts by the ocean. She greets me at the door with a little woolly monkey in her arms. The monkey is dressed in a simple pink pinafore with puffy sleeves. She makes no mention of the monkey and neither do I. Hilda has the unmistakable look of a Gypsy. But not your store-window bunko-squad, confidence-game variety. She is very sweet, sincere, and earnest. Inside the house are the healer's essentials: incense, crystals, candles, and spiritual Muzak. To my relief, she dismisses the monkey and leads me to a bright satin-covered futon where we discuss my hot flashes, vaginal dryness, night sweats, and lack of sleep.

Hilda has definite rules about sleep. "In the northern hemisphere it is proper to sleep with the head to the north, so that the magnetic currents flow parallel with the spine. In the southern hemisphere your head should be to the south and in the equatorial zone the head should be to the east. If you harmonize the direction of the flow of your own energies with the energies of the earth you will avoid conflict and achieve perfect sleep." I will try this when I get home.

Hilda felt that she could dim the flames of my flash through touch, prayer, and her special brand of healing energy. I was skeptical but what did I have to lose? She led me to a long table that was in the middle of the room. I got on it and lay down. She very slowly began passing her hands over my body, exploring my energy fields. She finds "jangling and buzzing" around my ovaries and throughout my entire reproductive system. She then summons the appropriate spirits into the room and fills them in on my problem. Once they were all briefed, she began the ritual. She laid her hands on my body and prayed to the patron saint of menopause and the spirits of night sweats, hot flashes, and vaginal dryness to relieve my symptoms, to unblock my energy, to free my channels, to heal me, to make me cool and wet. It was all very embarrassing but I wasn't going to hurt her feelings and besides, maybe it works. I know Lourdes does very well. I said to myself, Don't be such a cynic. Go with it. So I went with it. An hour later it was over.

An entranced Hilda then carefully washed my bad vibes and diseased energy off her hands with liquid Prell, opened a bottle of vintage holy water, and toasted the resurrection of my vagina. I got goose bumps like the ones you get when they sing the "Star-Spangled Banner." A half hour later I was flashing again. That night I discovered it wasn't practical to sleep with my head to the north. If I did my husband's feet would be in my mouth.

Hilda's therapy didn't work for me but it definitely wasn't life-threatening and there is something to the idea of releasing blocked energy. In fact, the release of blocked energy is an important part of several non-Western forms of healing, including the ayurvedic.

Ayurveda is the latest thing in ancient medicine. It is a system of healing from India that is 5,000 years old. When I arrive at the ayurvedic center I am expecting a very serene mystical environment with a matching mystic in long hair, beard, saffron robe, and sandals. When I enter the office, it is anything but serene. They are in the middle of an extensive remodeling—ladders, tools, Sheetrock, paint, plaster, and drop cloths fill a portion of what was once the waiting room. Inspecting the mess is the doctor. He is a very tall man with very short hair, more yuppie than Yogi, in suspenders, power tie, and buttondown. But he is shoeless. Is the reason religion or remodeling? I don't ask. He greets me in his stocking feet, hands together, palms facing each other, elbows away from his body like he is praying or meditating or about to crack his knuckles. He apologizes for the mess but explains that it is necessary so that he can give his patients the best possible care. "We are putting in a new Panchakarma therapy unit with a Swedena Shirodhara facility and a Udvartana." I nod, very impressed, although I have no idea what he is talking about.

He leads me to a bright modern office with light new beige carpeting, where he asks me to take off my shoes. Is the reason religion or the rug? Again I don't ask. I obediently take off my shoes and answer a lot of personal questions about hot foods, cold weather, my sex drive, dreams, attitude toward money, sleep habits, favorite foods, indigestion, digestion, and excretion.

He explains that this personal information helps him to diagnose my imbalances so that he can tailor a treatment to fit my body type. To find out what my body type actually is he has to take a pulse diagnosis—an ancient ayurvedic technique that will determine whether I am pitta, kapha, or vatta, the three forces or humors that control the mind and body. Pitta, which is fire, governs the digestive function; kapha, which is water, determines biological strength; and vatta, which is air, controls the nervous system and the process of elimination. When these life forces or doshas are balanced you get perfect health.

After taking a few minutes to read my pulse he has determined that I am a vatta type. Vatta is air but my hot flashes are pitta, which is fire. He decides to treat me not as a monodoshic vatta but as a bidoshic—a vatta/pitta with an emphasis on vatta. "Each person's treatment must be individual. That's the difference between ayurvedic and conventional medicine." Now that he has discovered my elemental imbalances he gives me a program that will restore my equilibrium and once again have my doshas living in harmony with each other.

I am wind-predominant so I have to take foods and choose a life-style that decreases the wind (vatta) dosha and increases the fire (pitta) and water (kapha) doshas. But I can't increase my fire dosha too much because that will feed my hot flashes. He recommends that I eat warm foods, oily food, and food with predominantly sweet, sour, and salty tastes. I am to avoid foods having predominantly pungent, bitter, or astringent tastes. He gives me a list of the foods that I can and cannot have.

He then tells me that I will need special ayurvedic herbs and minerals and teas, which he sells me. Finally, he writes out a detailed routine listing what I must do every day to get my doshas in balance. The daily routine includes "morning evacuation of bowels and bladder, oil massage to head, body, and soles of feet, herbal tea, gargle with sesame oil, and meditation." In the afternoon I'm to take a brief rest after my balanced pitta/vatta lunch and more meditation. Evening is more balanced food, aromatherapy, a relaxing walk, and early to bed. I am not allowed to work, read, stand, or watch TV during meals. I must not eat too quickly or too slowly, and the meals must be balanced so as to include all the tastes prescribed. I am to avoid ice-cold beverages and I am to drink a glass of hot water every hour. If I do this he assures me that my doshas will balance, I will achieve perfect health, and my dry vagina and hot flashes will disappear. I am to see him in a month to follow up on my progress.

This is a major commitment, a life-style, a full-time job. But I am ready to give it a try. I put on my shoes, go home, and follow his instructions to the letter. Whatever I did stirred up my vatta. I start to feel a Santa Ana blowing through my body. It grows from a gentle warm breeze to a super-hot, high-velocity powerful force that swirls around my insides. Before I know it, my doshas are out of control. My vattas and pittas and kaphas start dancing and dashing and prancing inside me with all the force and fury of a tornado. For some reason my air is feeding my fire and it is too much for my water. There is a major firestorm raging inside me and I can't stop it. Fire, air, and water pour from every orifice and I begin flashing every minute. I am jet-propelled. My humors are on a rampage and it is not funny. This is an ayurvedic emergency. I am having a dosha meltdown.

What have I done wrong? Did I feed my pitta and starve my vatta? Did I use too much sesame oil? Too little herb tea? Not enough meditation? Maybe all that hot water increased my vatta by decreasing my pitta or maybe I'm not even a vatta/pitta; maybe I have some kapha in me. Could I be tridoshic? I don't know. I am not an expert but I must talk to someone who is. There is no ayurvedic hotline and it is twenty-nine days to my next appointment. But I doubt if I can make it through another night like this. I immediately stop what I am doing and call the doctor. He is not in but I leave an urgent message on his machine and leave my delicate dosha balance alone until I hear from him.

Four days later the doctor calls me back. When I tell him about my night of 1,000 hot flashes he is ecstatic. "It's working! Your body house is being cleansed!" "Doctor, I am afraid my body house is gutted." I do not believe in pyrrhic victories. I had had enough. His theories might hold water but I couldn't. It was time to say *adios* to ayurveda.

After my ayurvedic experience I was a little timid about my next venture. I wanted to leave my doshas alone for a while so massage therapy seemed like a safe, harmless, logical choice. After talking with several New Agers I decided to try acupressure. Acupressure has its origins in ancient China. It basically uses the same techniques as acupuncture but instead of needles it uses fingertip pressure at specific points on the body to ease pain, calm anxiety, and provide relief from many ailments, including menopause.

My massage therapist, Joann, works in what I would describe as an "environment." When you enter her house, which doubles as her office, you hear the sounds of the jungle coming from concealed speakers and the oils she uses on your body fill the house and your senses with the wonderful smells of almond and vanilla and jasmine. The aromas are relaxing and stimulating and nothing like those heavy fragrances that come pouring out of fashion magazines and give you a headache.

Joann is a beautiful, ethereal young woman who lives in perfect harmony with three cats, a boyfriend, and a parakeet. Joann feels that she can help reduce the severity of my hot flashes, help me to sleep more soundly, and give me more energy. When I tell her I am all for this she has me lie down on a table, covers me with a sheet, and begins the therapy.

As she stimulates the pressure points she describes them. Each pressure point has a magical name and with her fingers she takes me through them like they are stops on some spiritual Orient Express. We go from Three Yin Crossing to Sinking Valley and Babbling Spring. We stop in Silk Bamboo Hollow and Middle Islet, change at Heavenly Pivot, continue on to Penetrating Valley, Very Great Abyss, Capital Bone, Yang Pond, and Cloud Gate, and wind up at the Extremity of Yin. It is a wonderful, energizing trip and when I leave I think maybe there is light at the end of the tunnel. Unfortunately, when I got home the light turned out to be just another hot flash.

The acupressure didn't stop my hot flashes, but after a few more sessions I did start to sleep better and have more energy. It also restored my confidence in alternative approaches to menopause. When I was once again in a "fearless state of mind" Joann suggested that I try reflexology, which she also practiced. The art of reflexology is based on the theory that certain areas of the feet are directly related to other parts of the body and by stimulating those body parts through the feet you can promote healing in the corresponding body part. It has been used successfully in helping both menopausal and menstrual problems. Having complete faith in Joann, I decided to put my feet in her hands but my heart was in my mouth.

THEY GOT THE WHOLE GAYLE IN THEIR HANDS

I lie down on a table and wince in pain as Joann uses the soles of my feet to get to the bottom of my problems. She holds my foot in her hand and plays with it like it's some kind of remote-control TV clicker, pressing points and switching channels with the speed and frequency of an impatient couch potato. We race through my body parts like they are programs on some space-age TV. We go from my heart to my lungs to my ovaries, back to my heart, and check out my liver. See what's going on in my kidneys, colon, bladder, and spleen. It is exciting but painful. The deep pressure required to turn on each body part is a major turnoff. Joanne tells me it only hurts the first time and that I will get used to it. But the pain gives me cold feet and the first time winds up being the last time. We agree that reflexology is not for me. Maybe acupuncture is. Joann suggests that I see an acupuncturist that she works closely with. "Try it and see what happens."

The acupuncturist lives and works in a neat little frame house. Inside, the house is Ethan Allen, not Ming Dynasty, and my acupuncturist, J. Scott Norton III, is Occidental, not Oriental. As he leads me to his office we walk past his wife and twin daughters who are juicing in the kitchen. After we spend an hour talking about my life-style and my emotions and my eating habits, he takes my pulse to determine my imbalances. Following a long careful read of my wrist he tells me that my kidney yin is off. In Chinese healing there are six "hollow" or yang organs and six "solid" or yin organs, of which the kidney is one. "There is too much fire in your kidney," he says. Since yin and yang and fire in the kidney are about as comprehensible to me as the theory of relativity, I remain silent as he tells me that by stimulating certain acupuncture points with needles he can balance my yin and yang, keep my meridians unblocked, and my life force or chi once again flowing freely.

I hate the idea of needles, even single-use disposable needles, but for now I am committed to an estrogen-free menopause. I close my eyes as he skewers my wrists and ankles with little needles. The needles give me a little jolt when they are inserted and once they are in I am aware of their presence. For the next twenty minutes I sit there like a human dart board as he explains the rest of the therapy.

J. Scott Norton III tells me that I am running out of kidney qi, which is my essence, which affects my sex drive and reproduction. Depleted kidney essence causes hot flashes, dry vagina, a loss of libido, and osteoporosis. "According to traditional Chinese medicine when a woman matures, there is a drop in essence, blood declines, and menopause occurs." Along with the acupuncture he prescribes herbs that will strengthen my kidneys and replenish my essence. They are cooked rehmannia, cornus, and ground dioscorea. He also prescribes herbs

THEY GOT THE WHOLE GAYLE IN THEIR HANDS

that contain estrogen-like compounds called phytoestrogens that will nourish my ovaries and adrenals. "They are a fraction as potent as estrogen and have no side effects when used correctly." These include licorice root, wild yam root, black cohosh, unicorn root, chaste berry, and dong quai, the king of the female complaint herbs. When he removes the needles I feel great. I am not sure whether this is because the needles were in or because they are now out.

For the next few months I have more holes put in me than a supermarket bulletin board. Along with the acupuncture, I take herbs in every shape, size, and form. I buy them fresh, dried, in tea leaves, tea bags, tinctures, capsules, and pills. I put them in drinks, on foods, and directly into my mouth. I nibble them, swallow them, and sniff them. I root for the roots and the needles but nothing works. For some reason they just can't clear my blocked meridians.

Scott the acupuncturist even tries a technique called moxibustion where he places an herb called moxa on a needle, ignites it, and puts it in an acupoint to stimulate the qi. It looks like a flaming herb shish kebob and is about as effective. It seems like the more needles he puts in me the more holes I have for my night sweats to seep out. Acupuncture and herbs have worked for thousands of years, but for some reason they weren't working for me. Besides the acupuncture, I was getting plenty of nee-

dling from my husband the cynic. It was all very dis-
couraging.

When I tell Scott how I'm feeling, he reminds me
that it takes time for the body to restore balance naturally. After another month we stop the herbs and acupuncture and try homeopathic medicine. Homeopathic
medicine is based on the principle that "like cures like."
The medicine contains minute doses of natural sub-
stances that in larger doses would produce the symptoms
they are used to treat. I am not sure how you bottle a hot
flash, but I will try it. For my hot flashes Scott prescribes
sepia, which is made from squid ink. The tablets are small
and white and round and don't work. Next I take them in
combinations—sulphur, lachesis, agnus, ignatia, cimic-
ifuga, and more sepia, sulphur, and lachesis. You do not
swallow homeopathic pills; you put them under your
tongue until they dissolve, and they do not dissolve
quickly. A side effect is short-term speech impairment,
which is caused when you try to talk while waiting for the
pills to dissolve. Unfortunately this is the only effect the
pills have on me. I continue to flash and sweat.

The combined efforts of acupuncture, herbs, home-
opathy, J. Scott Norton III, and me had little effect on my
essence, meridians, life force, yin and yang, and qi and
chi. I was taking it all very personally and so was he. I felt
bad that he felt bad and he felt bad that I felt bad that he
felt bad. When this happens it is time to move on even

though you feel bad that he will feel bad because you are moving on. But I will feel worse if I don't. So I did.

I had tried everything from age-old ayurveda, acupuncture, and herbs to New Age crystals and healing and aromatherapy, but nothing worked. When it was suggested that I try hypnotherapy, I flat-out refused. I had seen too many of those slick nightclub hypnotists on TV when I was a kid. I was not about to let some wise guy put me in a trance, and make me quack like a duck even if it might relieve my menopausal symptoms. Maybe it was time to wake up to the fact that my symptoms weren't going to go away naturally or holistically, that my choice was estrogen or nothing.

Just when I thought that I was out of options and my magical mystery tour had come to an end, a New Age New York friend of mine insisted that I see her nutritionist for my menopause. "The guy's a genius. He told me he never met a cancer patient who wasn't constipated." It didn't move me.

"That doesn't make him a genius," I said. When she told me he also said under no circumstances take estrogen, I asked her for his phone number. She hit an open nerve. I had to find out what this was all about.

I called his office the next day. He repeated to me what he told my friend. "Never take estrogen because it causes cancer." I asked him what I should take. He told me he wouldn't know until he analyzed my pubic hair.

Analyze my pubic hair? "Do I have to be there when you do it?" I asked nervously.

"Oh, no, just cut a healthy bunch off and send it in," he said matter-of-factly.

"Then what?" I asked matter-of-factly.

"When the results come back from the lab I'll analyze them and then we'll sit down and discuss it."

"I look forward to it," I said excitedly. That night I cut my pubic hairs, carefully avoiding the gray ones, put them in an envelope and sent it to him. You know, there's something very creepy about using the mails to transport pubic hair. I don't even know if it's legal. I would have much preferred sending my X rays.

About a month later I went to see him in his Upper Upper West Side office. I call it the Upper Upper West Side because once you got there you had to walk up four flights of stairs to get to his office. There were no magazines, there was no waiting room, but there were plenty of vitamins. Cartons were stacked everywhere. I felt like I was in the back of a vitamin truck.

Dr. Bemmelman, a very well-groomed, very healthy looking little man in his fifties, greeted me as I entered. He was the greatest-smelling man I had ever met. Very fresh, very natural, very healthy. As he led me around boxes of vitamins to his desk I couldn't help but think that Dr. Bemmelman, The Fragrance, could be a big seller or even Dr. Bemmelman, The Salad Dressing; I wasn't sure which one. Dr. Bemmelman asked me about my diet, my exercise regimen, and my medical history. He then opened up a folder and we got down to the serious business.

According to my pubic hair, I had too much calcium in my system, which he said could lead to arthritis and heart disease. He could tell by my look that I wasn't completely buying it. "Pubic hair doesn't lie," he said. He suggested that to reduce my calcium levels I cut out all dairy products and take certain supplements that he would supply and I would buy. I didn't want to reduce my calcium supplements because I was afraid of osteoporosis. When I told him my bone-density test was very high he said I had nothing to worry about. He assured me that if I followed his diet and vitamin regimen I would be in great shape, wouldn't get osteoporosis, and wouldn't suffer the effects of menopause. He was very convincing. I agreed to give it a try. As I left the office he introduced me to his dog, a very well-groomed, very healthy looking little poodle. She also smelled great and was a believer. "She eats my vitamins," he said proudly. The poodle looked about seven years old. That would be forty-nine in dog years. She looks pretty good for a dog that's going through menopause, I thought.

The next day the vitamins and the supplements arrived. There were so many boxes my doorman had to bring them up to my apartment on a dolly. Dr. Bemmelman prescribed a sodium selenite pill when I got up in the morning. After breakfast eighteen more pills: one vitamin B complex, one extra B_5 and one B_6, one vitamin E, one vitamin C, one L-cysteine, one bromelain, three iron, three zinc, one chromium, one magnesium, one echinacea, and two Fem-Tones, which contain ascorbic acid, dong quai, bioflavonoid, black cohosh, false unicorn root, licorice root, unicorn root, and fennel seed. After dinner I had to do it all over again. At bedtime I had to take two more Fem-Tones and one-quarter teaspoon of progesterone and vitamin E oil. I was to take another two Fem-Tones whenever I had menopausal symptoms. I was taking everything but WD-40. Things got so confusing that I swallowed the pills in alphabetical order just to be sure that I took them all. Usually your urine turns yellow from vitamins. Mine was neon. It glowed in the dark.

If you take vitamins in the doses I just described you have time for very little else. It's a bigger commitment than marriage or children. You spend most of your waking hours unscrewing and screwing, unpacking and packing, sorting and resorting, wrapping and rewrapping, ordering and reordering pills. Your house is taken over by tiny little bottles. They are everywhere—on shelves, in cabinets, behind furniture, in your refrigerator, in your closets, under your bed, in your pockets, in your purse, and on your mind. You are obsessed with them. It's all about A's and E's and D's and C's and B's and water and swallowing. It's no life and it's a no life that's very expensive. The costs were tougher to swallow than the pills—around $300 a month, and that's not counting the man-hours spent in the sorting, swallowing, and reordering phases.

For three weeks my menopausal symptoms completely disappeared. I was ecstatic. It was all worth it. The fourth week they returned. I was crushed. I called Dr. Bemmelman. He told me to continue my regimen and to increase the Fem-Tone. It didn't work. Taking all the pills was giving me diarrhea, making me lose weight, and getting me nauseated, and the expense was getting my husband even more nauseated. A few months later I gave up the program except for some vitamin E, C, and B complex. At the end of the year I took another bone-density test. It showed that I had lost some bone. I learned a valuable lesson from all of this. Don't listen to New Age friends, sweet-smelling nutritionists, or your pubic hair.

I had been searching everywhere for the Fountain of Youth when in fact it had been right under my nose in St. Augustine, Florida. That magical spring whose waters could bring eternal youth to all who drank and bathed in it is located not more than a couple of miles from where I live. This is the same spring that brought Ponce de León to St. Augustine in 1513 and me to it nearly five hundred years later.

The Fountain of Youth is located in a beautiful park near the ocean. A large statue of Ponce guards the spring. When you walk around the fountain on the lush green grass surrounded by ancient moss-laden magnolias you realize that our obsession with youth isn't new or particularly American. The Spanish were searching for it long before Elizabeth Arden, Estée Lauder, and Helena Rubinstein. Ponce de León didn't come to America looking for gold and spices and menopause. He came here looking for youth. It is in our blood and our genes. It is our heritage.

As I walk through the picnic area on my way to the gift shop where they sell the "youth" water I notice little children eating at the redwood picnic tables. Could these children be satisfied customers who came in cars and will go home in baby carriages? When I enter the gift shop the answer is obvious. All the clerks are in their sixties and look it. I buy a half gallon of the youth water anyway. I drink it all. It doesn't work. But we knew that.

Sex, Lies, and Menopause

The hormonal heat wave continues. In a single evening I experience more "hot wetness" than the heroine of a cheap romance novel. Unfortunately, my hot wetness is the result of hot flashes, not hot sex. In bed my husband no longer looks for my G-spot. Now he looks for a dry spot. The drop in estrogen levels has also caused my vaginal walls to become thin and dry, making sex painful. It's hard to decide which came first, not wanting to have sex or not wanting it because it hurt. Now sex has all the eroticism and pleasure of a full body wax. Except for the hot flashes there is absolutely no heat in our relationship. Birds do it. Bees do it. We don't. Menopause has had a magical effect on our sex life. It made it disappear. My vagina has become a vestigial structure. It is about as essential to my sex life as my appendix. Things have gotten so desperate that watching a Madonna video now qualifies as a sexual experience.

Sex had always been an important part of our marriage. We did it in place of, instead of, because of . . . We never needed a reason or an excuse or an occasion. Almost any problem could be worked out by me and my husband in bed. Sex used to solve problems; now it was the problem. Our lust had gone bust. Neither of us could get excited about sex and as a result we made love with the frequency of Halley's comet. Not too long ago we were having sex three times a week—now we were having sex no times a month. A multiple orgasm meant twice a year.

Surprisingly, this sexual drought didn't seem to bother my husband. He even kidded me about all the money we were saving on birth control and heating bills. My libido was shot and it appeared that his was also. We chose not to deal with our sexual problems. We found new ways to divert our sexual energy. The gym was a perfect place. We went seven days a week and did all our moaning and groaning and sweating and heavy breathing on the mats instead of the mattress. At night he went to bed with Ben-Gay and I went to bed with Oil of Olay. We drew comfort in the fact that the gym was going to add years to our life—long sexless years.

Another new passion was shopping. We spent a lot of time together malling. Plunging in and out of stores with wild abandon. Touching, grabbing, squeezing, and fondling the merchandise, lunging toward the counter, whipping out charge cards, making multiple purchases, screaming in ecstasy over a bargain, and moaning under the weight of our purchases.

When we went on vacation it used to be days and nights of sun and sex, mainly sex. Now it was days and nights of sun and shopping, mainly shopping. Nothing was more erotic than getting a 40 percent duty-free discount on a bottle of rum or a Swiss watch. We came home tired, tan, and satisfied.

He knew what pleased me and I knew what pleased him. We became less and less romantic and more and more pragmatic. For Valentine's Day I used to get sexy underwear and expensive perfume. Now I got cash. For our anniversary it used to be a candlelight dinner, wine, and flowers. This time we stayed home, turned down the lights, got undressed, jumped into bed, and after a marathon session of TV watching ordered a juicer and a laptop computer from the Home Shopping Network.

In bed, we purged any sexual urges with new obsessions. "Is that your hair on the pillow or mine?" "Was that sound coming from your stomach or mine?" "I'm not snoring, you are."

In the good old days nothing got in the way of sex. Now sex got in the way of nothing. I'd say "Want to make love?" and not mean it. He'd say "Yes" and not mean it, and by the time we got to the bedroom we both prayed that something would stop us. Anything. A fight over his having left the toilet seat up, or the temperature of the bedroom, or "Is the door locked?" were all sure 100-percent-guaranteed sex stoppers. In bed we would get passionate over who got to turn on the TV and fondle the remote-control clicker. If this kept up, we would soon be sleeping in bunk beds and it would be curtains for our marriage.

We were building to a crisis. My problem was my menopause. Was his problem our marriage? Why did he make no demands on me sexually? Why was his penis on hold? Was I no longer attractive? Did he want children I couldn't bear? He told me that a healthy man can father children as long as he lives, but it was over for a woman at menopause. I thought it was very insensitive of him. I tried to ignore it but I couldn't. I told him he hurt me and made me feel very insecure. He told me he didn't mean anything by it and not to worry. I wasn't worried. I was hysterical! Now that I couldn't have children maybe he'd want some high-heeled, miniskirted, nubile young thing with enough eggs to populate a major city to bear his progeny.

Is he no longer attracted to me now that I am without eggs and out of the labor force? Have I joined the ranks of that gray, nonreproductive, faceless middle-aged mass? Have I faded away like some old soldier? Have I become sexually invisible? The next time I look in a mirror will no one look back? My confidence is gone. Now when I sit in a restaurant having lunch and a man looks in my direction I wonder if he's looking at me or what I'm eating. Is he picturing me with my clothes off or is he having fantasies about my salad dressing? I am a middle-aged, married, menopausal woman with hot flashes, a dry vagina, and no libido and yet I would like this total stranger to be as hungry for me as he is for my sandwich. I refuse to become an invisible middle-aged woman.

What do I do? Do I act my age or not act my age? Do I dress like Madonna or Barbara Bush? Am I Cher or Queen Elizabeth? I want to remain a person and have my own identity. I don't want to go through the rest of my life feeling that I lost my wallet with everything in it.

I am paranoid. Now that our sex life has gone belly up and I am sexually invisible I bet my husband has found himself some twenty-year-old named Jennifer or Melissa or Heather. Men do strange things at midlife. First they act like babies. Next they go out with them. They don't want to grow up and get old. In their search to find themselves and stay young, judges leave the bench to become stand-up comedians and clowns leave the circus to become congressmen. Others join the men's movement. They go off on wilderness weekends with nothing but an ax and a cellular phone, hoping that crying and dancing and drumming and male bonding will help them find the wild man within them and revitalize their gonads. Still others leave their wives, start dating their son's girl-friends, and appear on Oprah during sweeps.

For some reason middle-aged men think it is not

gravity but their wives who are responsible for the drop of their penises and the death of sex. They think that a new, younger lover will resurrect their body and their sex life. To prepare for this second coming they cap their teeth, dye their hair, pierce their ears, and open their shirts, waiting for that moment when they can trade in the old wife and wagon for a young mistress and a new motorcycle. Somehow they believe that sex with a young woman will take their minds off prostates and Pritikin. That Guns N' Roses will bring back their gums n' regularity.

Will my husband become another midlife-crisis cliché? So far I see no overt signs of hormonal hysteria. He is not taking any outrageous fashion risks and he does not appear to be cheating. He doesn't shave, shower, and mousse before he takes out the garbage, and after taking out the garbage he doesn't return five hours later smelling of motel soap. But that doesn't mean a thing. A friend of mine who thought that she was happily married to her dentist husband was rudely awakened when he got up one morning screaming "It's all about teeth!" and ran off to Oregon with a cocktail waitress to make sandals and "find himself."

If my husband must find himself, that's okay. He'd just better not find himself with another woman because if I find him with another woman he's going to find himself without a wife. In the state I'm in I'm not about to confront him because if it's true I really don't know what

I'll do. I used to have all the answers. Now all I have is questions. I don't want to share my paranoia with my friends but I've got to talk to someone. Not anyone. A woman. A wise woman. My neighbor Karen, who just had her baby delivered naturally at home, suggested that I talk to her midwife. "She's seen it all," Karen says. I was under the impression that midwives were a thing of the past, like movie theater matrons, mah-jongg players, and flat-chested models. Maybe it is time to see a midwife at midlife.

My image of a midwife is someone who comes to your house on a buckboard, wears a bonnet, and tells you to tear up sheets and boil water. To my surprise the modern midwife has her own office, drives a Volvo, is state-licensed, and wears a beeper. When you meet Tina, you know instantly that she is a midwife. She was born to midwife. She is caring and knowing. Tina is in her forties but a part of her is still in the '60s. She wears a flower in her hair, a long dress, and has the spirituality of a love child. It's very hard to talk about your sex life with a stranger, but from the minute I meet her, Tina is a friend. When I tell her I'm not pregnant but menopausal, a '60s "Wow" pops out of her mouth.

She patiently listens as I tell my sad tale of man's inhumanity to woman and the decline and fall of his penis and our sex life. When I am finished she assures me that I am not the only married woman in North America having no sex and no desire. Many postnatal women have similar problems, and birth and babies and menopause have comparable psychological and physical effects on women and their relationships. In both you are at the mercy of your hormones.

When Tina talked about loss of libido, painful sex, low self-image, dry vagina, wild mood swings, hormones on a rampage, hair growing in strange places, discolored skin, hair loss, crankiness, irritability, blues, incontinence, and sleepless nights she wasn't talking about menopause; she was talking about childbirth. The more she described the physical and psychological effects of pregnancy and birth the more I could identify with the pregnant woman. They had babies, I had hot flashes. Except for the baby shower and stretch marks the effect was pretty much the same. Both keep you up all night, and make you tired and cranky and uninterested in sex. Both consume your life and your thoughts to the exclusion of your husband. Your obsession with them and attention to them causes resentment and anger and no sex.

Tina tells me that my husband's probably feeling replaced and jealous and tired and lonely and left out. That he's probably shell-shocked from the hot flashes, the night sweats, the wet bed, the sleepless nights, and my lack of libido. "A little while ago you were an aphrodisiac and now you are saltpeter," she says. She is absolutely right. Wet beds and dry vaginas and sleepless nights would numb any man's gonads. And even if he could get past all that and still want to make love, I made him feel like sex gave me all the pleasure of slamming my finger in a car door.

When Tina suggests that maybe I was too focused on my own needs to the exclusion of my husband's, it really hits home. I realize that since my first hot flash it's been all about me and my menopause. In the last year I have talked about little else. I have been in a menopause coma, completely out of it and oblivious to my husband's needs. I never ask him about his day or his work or his anything. I do not have a clue about what's going on in his brain. We hardly talk and when we talk it's about me . . . me . . . me! My hormones have made a cuckold of my husband. He is playing second fiddle to a hot flash and a dry vagina.

I feel so guilty. If he is having an affair with one of those midlife-crisis groupies I would understand. I would understand but under no circumstances would I stand for it. Tina calms me down by telling me that birth and menopause are a time of change and an opportunity to grow. "Your sex life and your marriage don't have to end at menopause. This doesn't have to be a crisis without a solution. You are not a victim. Take charge." When I ask her if my husband is punishing me for my menopause, she reminds me that she is not a marriage counselor. When I tell her that she could be another Dr. Ruth, she smiles and changes the subject. She tells me she will show me how she helps new mothers bring life back to the bedroom after they have given birth.

"Have you ever kegeled?" "Is it like the samba?" I ask half-seriously. She laughs and tells me it is not a dance but a pelvic-floor exercise that is excellent for strengthening vaginal muscles, and was originally developed to prevent urinary incontinence in mothers after birth. I do not have this problem but Tina recommends the kegel exercise for other reasons. "Keeping all the muscles surrounding your internal organs toned and tight will prevent excessive dryness and fallen organs." It is also supposed to relax you and make sex more gratifying.

There is no Jane Fonda kegel tape, no Nautilus kegel machine. It can be done with just you and your sphincter. To kegel, all you have to do is imagine that you want to stop urinating and squeeze the sphincter muscles in your vaginal area firmly. Practice this squeeze technique while counting to three, then relax.* The nice thing about kegeling is that you don't need an outfit or a gym or even sneakers. You can do it anytime anywhere anyplace as long as you don't do it with a full bladder. I can sit on a bus or talk to my clergyman or chat with my neighbors and I could be kegeling my brains out and nobody would know the difference. A hundred or so of these totally

*See Notes.

undetectable exercises daily can do wonders for your vagina and your sex life.

For a new mother the estrogen levels drop dramatically in the first six weeks after delivery. Also, lactation causes the vagina to be dry and sensitive and makes sex very painful. In a menopausal woman, as the estrogen levels drop the same thing happens, only the vagina becomes smaller, especially in a woman who hasn't had any children. For this, Tina recommends natural lubricants like olive, wheat germ, and sesame oils. She doesn't recommend foams. "Foam is for emergency landings and runways, not vaginas." Other don'ts are Vaseline (it is water-soluble) and oil that contains alcohol. As Tina describes the natural vaginal toppings and dressings I can't help but get the feeling that when you put all this stuff on, it's less like making love and more like making a salad. My biggest fear is that after we make love and I ask, "Was it good for you, honey?" my husband will say, "Needs a little more oregano." For my vaginal itching Tina recommends oatmeal baths: "Just put some cooked oatmeal in a strainer and hold it under the tap as you fill the tub." I will give it a try but I am afraid that it's going to take a lot more than salad dressing and breakfast cereal to make my sex life more appetizing. Sensing that I am a little discouraged, Tina tells me that nothing is forever. Not morning sickness or night sweats or hot flashes.

I point out that pregnancy and morning sickness don't last more than nine months, while menopause and hot flashes can last more than nine years. Tina tells me that feeling sorry for myself isn't going to accomplish anything. I must deal with the problem. The most important thing is to do the thing I'm not doing. "Talk about it. When you get home ask him about his day. How he feels and then listen, really listen."

After Tina has helped me give birth to my menopause she boils water for herb tea and we sit in her homey little office and reminisce. As we get into it we discover that we have something in common. In the summer of 1969, Tina and I and about 400,000 of our contemporaries went to Woodstock. Tina remembers it as being a "definitely happening experience." Tina was a love child, the real thing. She was naked and free and part of the Woodstock generation. I was just a tourist in bell bottoms and a vest. It was twenty-one years, 252 periods, and one menopause ago but I'll never forget it. Three days of hair, rain, dirt, mud, music, and excruciating menstrual cramps. It was wonderful. It's hard to believe that this child of the '60s has become the menopausal woman of the '90s. That I am now just another aging Aquarian who has recently dropped out of reproduction to do my own thing, only now my "thing" is menopause.

It seems like a big leap from Woodstock to menopause. From Hippy to Yippy to Preppy to Yuppy to atrophy. In truth nothing has changed. When I was at Woodstock twenty-something years ago I felt unsure and powerless and out of control. I was trying to figure it all out and I still am. It took me the first forty-something years of my life to learn how to deal with men and sex. Now that I am at the point where I can put all my wisdom to good use I am betrayed by my hormones. I got so caught up in the care and feeding of my menopause that I forgot about my femininity and my relationship. I was married to my menopause. That was my universe. Some universe. Not exactly the stuff of Big Bangs. This is a very trying time but I will try anything to get through it. Now that I am aware of the problem I will deal with it. I feel awful but a lot better.

When I get home I do one hundred kegels, take a deep breath, and then ask my husband, "How was your day and are you having an affair?" To which he replies, "No." "Then what are you doing with your penis?" I ask. "Right now my penis is not a priority," he answers. This is hard to believe. "You mean to tell me that if an eighteen-year-old cheerleader bounced naked into this bedroom and wanted to do it with you, you wouldn't get aroused?" There is a long pause. We are now in a gray area. I quickly move on. "What I mean is, do you look at other women?" "Sure, I look at other women. I just can't see them very clearly anymore. When you hit fifty the whole world is small print, including women." I press on. "So you are not cheating."

"How could I cheat? My memory is so bad now that if a woman gave me her phone number I couldn't remember it and even if I wrote it down my eyesight is so bad that I couldn't read it and even if I was lucky enough to read it and remember it I'd be so afraid of getting a heart attack from an overdose of sexual gratification that I would just lie there limply, wondering what I was doing in this strange bed in the first place."

"Have you lost your sex drive?" "I don't think I lost it. I think I misplaced it. When you are preoccupied with your age and your heart and your flab and your hair and your career, you don't spend much time thinking about the care and feeding of your penis. You want to leave it alone, don't get it too excited. There are too many other things to worry about. I am more interested in getting up than in getting it up." When I ask him how my menopause affected him he tells me that my hot flashes and night sweats and dry vagina did not exactly make him feel young and virile and immortal. "I was trying to ignore my middle age and you were reminding me of it every day. I learned a lot about me by looking at you. But I was not resentful and I was definitely not having a midlife crisis." "So you're okay," I say. "I didn't say that. Right now I'm not worried about losing my hair or my memory or my teeth or even an erection. I'm worried about losing my life. All I have to do is look around me and I see guys my age falling like flies." He reminds me that the life

like this happen?' 'He was so young.' There were even conspiracy theories. Was the Stairmaster the lone assassin or did it have help in killing him? It was agreed that it was not just the Stairmaster that killed him. It was helped by things like work, ambition, and the hormonal hysteria of middle-aged men trying to prove that they are still bigger and better and stronger than the next guy.

"Men have this need at middle age to find themselves. Unfortunately, Mel Franklin found himself dead. His last words were, 'Call my office and tell them I'll be late.' The late Mel Franklin died on the way to the hospital. The next day the young lions all but forgot it. Their locker-room talk quickly returned to heated discussions over the value of instant replay, the importance of cleavage, and the wisdom of the designated hitter rule. When someone asked what happened to Mel one of them casually dismissed it with 'Some old guy died.' Some old guy?! I'm three years older than that 'some old guy.' I was shaken but they remained unruffled and immortal. In fact, they had taken the firing of a good-looking young female aerobics instructor much harder than the death of Mel Franklin. They continued loading large slabs of weight on the Nautilus machines and pumping massive amounts of iron as if nothing had happened. The older lions, myself included, took it much harder. We personalized it. We had gotten our middle-age wake-up call. We realized that death is a fact of life. There but for the grace of a few extra push-ups could be us. It could happen straining to open a jar of pickles or chasing a cab, and no amount of aerobics, oat bran, or vitamin supplements is going to stop it. Death is the real midlife crisis. The rest is kid's stuff. We all chipped in and sent his family a big bouquet of 'Thank God it isn't us' flowers and in two days it was business as usual except none of us older guys went on that Stairmaster again.

"Since Mel's death every little ache has a sinister meaning. A headache is a tumor, heartburn is a cardiac. Misplacing the car keys is Alzheimer's. My body is out to kill me and I have to be on guard. I am no longer worried about life passing me by. Now I am worried about a bypass. I am no longer preoccupied with finding myself. All I care about is not finding myself dead. I used to worry about dings on my car and bad haircuts and moving up a few tax brackets. Now I worry about the tingling in my kidney, the throb in my temple, and the beat of my heart. I worry about how much of my carotid artery all that cheesecake I used to eat blocked and what did my great-grandfather die of and is it genetic? Now what's good for my head is not to get a brain tumor. At this point loss of libido and impotence is not important. It's hard to get hard when you're worried about rigor mortis. When your own mortality is getting you down it's hard to get it up."

When I asked him why he didn't share this with me he said that he had made a halfhearted attempt, but I was preoccupied with my hot flashes and he was having trouble facing it himself. When I asked him why he didn't talk to his friends or the other men in the gym about it, he told me that men don't share secrets and that they don't face things head-on the way women do. "You are up front about your menopause. You share it with me and your friends—even with total strangers. Men aren't like that. We face middle age and our own mortality the way we face everything else that makes us vulnerable—with denial or excess or excuses or aggression. I couldn't talk to the guys about it because no one would have been honest, including me. Men just don't tell the truth about business or the bedroom or their insecurities. They tell fish stories to prove that they are supermen. Since puberty I have been exaggerating the length of my penis, the number of conquests, and the frequency of orgasms. As a kid I routinely lied about eight-orgasm evenings, followed by four-orgasm mornings. And going 'all the way' with everyone. In my fish stories none got away.

"If I told the guys of my recent limp libido they would have made me feel like I was all alone. When in truth, at this stage of our lives all of us would have to chip in for an erection. When it comes to your penis you don't give or get straight answers."

I am overwhelmed by his openness and honesty and pain. I am underwhelmed by my recent insensitivity and self-involvement. For the first time in a long time our relationship is coming into focus. Those jokes he made about birth control and sex were really just a defense against his own insecurities and loss of libido. For him, my lack of desire wasn't a frustration; it was a relief. Now that I was listening I realized that he, too, was experiencing the same anxiety and insecurity that I was. He, too, realized he was getting older, and my experiences made him come face-to-face with his own vulnerability and mortality. He wanted to minimize his middle age. I magnified it. He wanted to ignore it. But I kept reminding him. He talked about kids at old age so he wouldn't think it was over. He watched Mets games not because he was a baseball fan but because they revived his youth. I reminded him that he was getting old. I wasn't experiencing menopause. We were experiencing menopause.

We had to work this out. We were definitely not in lust but we wanted to stay together and do something about our dear departed sex life. That night we went out for a romantic dinner and when we came home we went directly to bed and had a passionate discussion about how to fix our busted libidos. We both came to the conclusion that during these sexual hard times the thing to do was not to replace but to fix and remodel what we had spent ten years together building.

We began by buying a bunch of women's magazines that had articles about how to put the "sizzle" back in your sex life. One suggested that I buy erotic playthings

IS IT HOT IN HERE OR IS IT ME?

like crotchless lace bodystockings, naughty nighties, pistachio pasties, and pineapple panties. Unfortunately, sexual edibles are an acquired taste that even in my sex-starved state I just do not have the stomach for. Another magazine suggested that we spice up our foreplay by renting erotic movies. After visiting our local video store and self-consciously reading the descriptions on the boxes for *Monumental Knockers, Volume II* and *Sperm Busters*, we left with *Fried Green Tomatoes.*

In one magazine a sex therapist advised fantasies and role playing—if I dressed as a nurse or a pizza waitress it would be the ultimate turn-on. Still another said I could heat up his hormones by slipping him notes like "You have a date in the shower in half an hour; clothes optional." There was no shortage of articles and theories and tips on how to put the fire back in your loins. It seems that loss of libido is a very hot topic. But although the advice is well-intentioned, after all was said and done my husband and I would have a great deal of trouble doing this stuff with a straight face.

I am afraid that for us no amount of leather and chains, arousal lotions and love potions, lubricating oils and ecstasy coils, sex ploys or erotic toys is going to take the place of some good old-fashioned rubbing and touching and clutching.

At this point I wasn't interested in vaginal, clitoral, or multiple orgasms. I was interested in painless sex. I had tried everything but Novocain. I even tried Tina's vaginal dressings. They relieved the pain but they required too much preparation. We needed more spontaneity for our combustion. It was time once again to see a doctor. I predict the scenario. He will inspect my cervix, make some noises, take some notes, explain to me what a hot flash feels like, and write me off with a prescription for estrogen. I go and he does. I am unwilling to take the estrogen pill—comprehensive HRT—so he prescribes estrogen cream, which is applied vaginally every other day. With it I am to take progesterone pills ten days out of every month, which are supposed to remove the risk of uterine cancer.

Before I filled the prescription I thought carefully about my alternatives. There were none. I know that estrogen has potential side effects, but so does no sex. Within a few weeks I felt the effects of the estrogen cream. There was no pain and we started to have sex again.

Whoever said "No pain, no gain" wasn't talking about our sex life. My only fear is that with all the estrogen my husband is coming in contact with he'll develop huge breasts. My husband isn't worried. He says huge breasts are a small price to pay for feeling like a man again.

The Heart of the Matter

Every year salmon swim upstream to spawn, the swallows return to Capistrano, and my husband and I visit my in-laws in south Florida. We join thousands of other snowbirds on their annual migration back to the land of the empty nester and the early-bird special. This little guilt trip had always been fun except for this year. The year of menopause and midlife crisis and my mother-in-law's heart attack.

The attack caught us all by surprise. It was the cardiac equivalent of Pearl Harbor. No one expected my mother-in-law to get a heart attack. Women don't get heart attacks! We were wrong. Dead wrong. The fact is more than 500,000 American women die of cardiovascular disease each year. Women get as many heart attacks as men; they just get them a little later. By age fifty-five it's our number-one killer. Researchers believe that estrogen boosts the level of HDL, the good cholesterol that helps keep the arteries clear and unclogged. After menopause, when estrogen levels decline, its protection is lost and the risk of heart attack and stroke increases dramatically.

When women do have heart attacks, they are twice as likely as men to die within the first few weeks. One of the reasons for this is that they often fail to get thorough and prompt medical attention because of the widespread notion that they are at less risk than men. Nearly one-third of all heart attacks in women go undiagnosed because the victim mistakes the symptoms for something else. My mother-in-law was one of those women.

Es, like most women, had a mortal fear of breast cancer. She examined her breasts regularly, saw her doctor every six months, and had a yearly mammogram. She was totally focused on her breasts and paid no attention whatsoever to her heart, even though the chances of her dying from a heart attack were more than double that of dying from cancer of any kind. She totally ignored the risk factors that put her in danger for a heart attack. What's worse, so did her doctor.

When Es started getting chest pains she thought it was heartburn. Her doctor concurred. If she had been a man she would have been referred to a cardiologist for more tests. Instead she was referred to the pharm-fresh section of her supermarket for more Maalox. This diagnosis is not uncommon. Until recently, all the male medical community knew about a woman's heart was that you sent a card on Valentine's Day. In the past, all heart research completely bypassed women and focused on men. True, Es's doctor wasn't a cardiologist, but he didn't have to read her EKG to know she was at risk. All he had to do was read her shopping list. It was deadlier than a Lucrezia Borgia cookbook. If he had spent a little time asking Es about her life-style and less time learning how to spell sphygmomanometer he would have seen the handwriting on the walls of her arteries and known that her cardiac was about to arrest her.

My in-laws were nutritional underachievers. They lived in lipid-land. They were thirty pounds overweight and each had the caloric intake of a sumo wrestler. They consumed cream by the quart, butter by the tub, cheese by the pound, antacid by the gallon, and their diet contained more salt than the Dead Sea. They thought ketchup was a vegetable and ice cream health food (because of the calcium). They ate their apples in strudel, their oranges in cakes, and their bananas in splits. Everything was deep-fried, floating in sauce, swimming in cheese, and bathed in butter. Es knew cholesterol was bad for you but she had her magic bullet. She had her oat bran. All the oat bran hype had led her to believe that a couple of muffins and a bowl of cereal would dislodge the daily accumulation of sludge that was clogging the walls of her arteries. Somehow she thought that the oat bran, like a roll of super-strength Bounty, would soak up the fat and gristle and take it away. So she kept eating like there was no tomorrow, and there almost wasn't.

The fat and the grease and the gristle built to a point where she had arterial gridlock at the intersection of aorta and vein and she had a heart attack. Fortunately, she recovered. But we still are nervous. Because 39 percent of women who have a heart attack will die within a year, and even if they survive the first year they are twice as likely to have a second attack. These facts alone are enough to give you a heart attack.

This is our first visit since Es got out of the hospital and I'm looking forward to it with the same enthusiasm that I would to a mammogram. I am expecting the worst. It's true that whenever we call she assures us that she's fine but that doesn't mean anything. My mother-in-law isn't a complainer. All her life she has cooked, cleaned, shopped, and menopaused without a complaint. When she had her kidney stones not a word. Painful gum surgery—not a whimper. She's the kind of person who could get brain surgery in the morning, take two aspirins, wax the floors, clean the oven, prepare a meal for twelve, and never say a word. This time I expected to find her in bed, inactive, and in bad shape. I was in for a big surprise.

They both looked great. The last time I had seen Es she was in bed noshing from an I.V. bottle and my father-in-law, Irv, was badly out of shape. His waist had gotten so high that he looked like he was being swallowed by his trousers. I definitely would not use the word "vital" in describing them. This time when I tell them that they look great, I mean it. They have obviously made some serious life-style changes in the six months since our last visit. Es had completed a twelve-week cardiac rehabilitation program given at the hospital that included exercise, diet, nutrition, and life-style counseling. After proudly displaying her newly laminated "Healthy Heart Club" certificate she led me into the kitchen where everything you need to know about diet, nutrition, and your heart was neatly placed under cute little magnets on the door of the refrigerator. There were dietary guidelines from the American Heart Association, the latest health news and low-fat recipes from magazines and newspapers, big articles, small clippings, long handwritten lists and short typed ones. This was no longer a refrigerator door; this was now a nutritional kiosk. Es tells me that keeping it current is a full-time job. Because the rules are always changing: "One day shrimp is bad, the next day it's good. What's good today can kill you tomorrow. It changes so fast you can get whiplash."

In the past, the contents of her refrigerator had broken every known law of nutrition. Now it had the Good Heartkeeping Seal of Approval. The refrigerator that was once Adipose Alley was now Health Central. Inside, it was better stocked than her medicine chest. Gone were the widow makers—the bacon and sausage, the pickled herring and cream sauces, the sour cream and dips, the salt-filled breads, meats, and dairy products. In their place were fat-free or fat-reduced nutritional knockoffs like plain low-fat yogurt and water-packed tuna and fresh fruits and vegetables. It was obvious that Es no longer had any intention of dying off the fat of the land.

Dinner that night was light years away from the cholesterol-clogged days of the past. The traditional homecoming meal was usually eggplant parmesan, a calorie-laden, heart-stopping time bomb that was drowned in eggs, fried in oil, smothered in cheese, embalmed in meat sauce, entombed in bread crumbs, and buried in salt. It was usually served with plenty of bread and butter, followed by ice cream and cake, antacid and TV, and stacks of snacks and munching and crunching until the playing of the "Star-Spangled Banner" marked the end of both the programming and partaking day. This ritual had now been replaced by a newer streamlined, slim-downed version of the cardiac special. The new parmesan had one-third the calories and almost no fat. Es broiled instead of deep-frying, used fat-free cheese, cut out the meat, used just egg whites, and made it almost fat-free. There was no bread and butter and for dessert we had angel food cake, which surprisingly enough has no fat and no cholesterol. My mother-in-law got her new eggplant parmesan recipe from *Prevention* magazine. She used to get her old ones from the back of meat sauce and mayonnaise jars. Es had learned how to prepare food that tastes good in a way that won't kill you. The meal was low in fat and high in taste.

Later, while we were putting things away in the kitchen, Es gave me the lowdown on calories, cholesterol, and fat. The desirable cholesterol level for healthy adults is 200 or less. Above that you increase your risk of heart problems. Get above 250 and you've got a date with an angel. Es is aiming to keep her cholesterol level below 180, which for her is the acceptable level. She believes that if you do it right you can keep your cholesterol level below 200 just by diet and exercise alone, without the use of drugs. The idea is to keep dietary fat intake to below 30 percent of your daily calories, and no more than 10 percent of your daily calories should come from *saturated* fat.

Everybody worries about cholesterol, but the real killer is saturated fats. These fats have not only been linked to heart disease but to cancer as well. They are found in animal, dairy, and meat by-products, and in coconut, palm, and palm kernel oils. If you eat too much saturated fat and cholesterol, the "bad" cholesterol (LDL) can increase in the bloodstream, you build plaque on your artery walls, and you are headed for a run-in with your heart. To keep the "bad" cholesterol down (below

130) and the "good" (HDL) up (between 50 and 60) you have to limit the consumption of foods high in saturated fat and limit your cholesterol intake to below 300 mg a day. For every 1 percent cut in cholesterol we get a 2 percent drop in heart-disease risk.

As she goes into further detail about the good HDL and its evil sister LDL I nod my head like I'm interested, but in truth this information is drier than a package of rice cakes. I want specifics. I want information that I can use everyday. Es gives me specifics. The average menopausal woman with a daily caloric intake of 1,800 calories should not eat more than 60 mg of fat a day and no more than 20 of these milligrams should come from satu-rated fat. Unfortunately, this is easier said than done. To determine the actual fat grams in a given meal you'll need a calculator, a metric scale, and a 5,000-page food-composition handbook. To determine the calories and grams of fat per serving, multiply the fat grams by 9 (the calories in each gram of fat), divide by the calories per serving, and multiply by 100. This new information is harder to digest than a bowl of dry fiber. What Es fails to realize is that I'm mathematically illiterate. I can't bal-ance my checkbook; how am I going to balance my diet? I can't understand a Hammacher-Schlemmer catalog; how am I going to read a food-composition book? I don't want every meal to be April 15 and I don't want to have to take my accountant every time I go shopping.

Es tells me to forget the figuring and just cut down on all fat. If you lower your fat intake to 20–25 percent of total calories you'll automatically cut down your saturated fat intake because about one-half the fat we eat is saturated. Es had figured out a way to do this. She studied labels, read magazines and newspapers, books and brochures, and made a list of things to do and remember that would, without a doubt, keep you well within the American Heart Association dietary guidelines. She very carefully broke down all her fat-cutting tips into little easy-to-swallow bite-sized bits of fat-fighting, lipid-licking, triglyceride-trouncing information. If I stuck to her guidelines I wouldn't have to worry. She then removed a well-worn handwritten list from the refrigerator door and handed it to me. Es is a great believer in lists. Lists are an important part of her life. She even talks with a list. She always has three reasons for this and five reasons for that, and now she has a list to attack fat:

ES'S TOP 10 WAYS TO CUT FAT AND AVOID INTENSIVE CARE

1 *Avoid completely tropical oils* (saturated fats) like coconut oil, palm oil, and palm kernel oils, and other saturated fats like butter.

2 *Go easy on the good oils* (monosaturated fats) like olive oil and canola oil. They may be good for your heart but

they are bad for your *waist*. They have the same fat calories as the bad oil. There are 120 fat calories in just one tablespoon of oil no matter whether it's saturated or unsaturated. Just four tablespoons of any oil use up your daily limit for fats.

3 *Stay away from processed meats* like sausage, bologna, salami, and hot dogs. Seventy to 80 percent of their total calories come from fat. Even a "low-fat" sausage still gets 60 percent of its calories from fat.

4 *Limit yourself to one* three-and-one-half-ounce portion of lean meat (fish, chicken, etc.) per day. That portion is roughly the size of a deck of cards. Trim away fat. Just by removing the skin from a chicken breast you can cut the fat calories in half. Stay away from "choice" and "prime" cuts. Choose "select," which has less fat. Avoid duck and goose and pre-basted turkeys.

5 *Go easy on cheeses,* which are often fattier than meat. Go easy on eggs. One large egg yolk contains almost the entire daily allowance for cholesterol (250–275 mg.). An egg white contains no cholesterol and is a good source of protein.

6 *Choose low-fat or no-fat* dairy products. If you drink two glasses of whole milk every day for a year, it will give you about twelve pounds of dietary fat. But two glasses of skim milk every day for a year will provide less than a tenth of a pound of fat.

7 *Stay away from mayonnaise.* It is 99 percent fat with a little egg yolk, which is 99 percent cholesterol. Eat foods that reduce cholesterol level—salmon, sardines, tuna, green vegetables, and soybean oil.

8 *Do not fry anything.* A baked potato is 100 calories; french-fry it and it is 300. Invest in nonstick cookware and use an aerosol cooking spray.

9 *Go easy on salt.* The American Heart Association recommends no more than 3,000 mg a day (one teaspoon has 2,132 mg). Rinse anything canned under water to remove most of the salt. Eat plenty of potassium; it helps remove the salt from your system. (Bananas, papaya, lima beans, cantaloupe, prunes, peaches, and orange juice are all potassium-rich.)

10 *Learn how to read food labels.* When I ask Es how to read them, she tells me she'll teach me when we go shopping.

That night I fell asleep counting saturated fats and cholesterol. The next morning when I got up I ran into Es standing in the kitchen in tights and sneakers like some kind of Grandma Jock. "How do I look? I never look in the mirror. If I did I'm afraid I'd never leave the house."

I tell her she looks great and admire her new Rockports. She tells me she walks for an hour every day. Doctor's orders. "He told me it's good for osteoporosis, my weight, raises my good cholesterol, and just by walking thirty minutes every day you can reduce your risk of dying from heart disease by 50 percent." He also said that not walking is as dangerous as smoking and high cholesterol. I ask her if she ever exercised before. "Never. Never even owned a pair of sneakers. I walked a little but I never considered that exercise. It was transportation." In fact, she thought exercise was bad for your heart, that being inactive was still the best way to avoid a heart attack. "Everyone we knew who got a heart attack got it chasing a bus or shoveling snow or climbing stairs. Every time we read the paper there would be a story about somebody who died of a heart attack jogging so they wouldn't die of a heart attack."

We both put on suntan lotion with an SPF the equivalent of aluminum siding and I join her as she goes for her walk. When we reach the supermarket Es gives me a crash course in label reading. The language appears to be English but when you try to make sense of it, it is harder to decipher than the Rosetta Stone. Labelese is semi-comprehensible jargon designed to confuse the shopper. Food labels have less credibility than a supermarket tabloid and are as carefully regulated as professional wrestling. "Truth in labeling" is an oxymoron and only a complete moron would believe some of the claims made on many food products. New laws requiring easier-to-read labels should change some of this in the near future, but until then it's buyer beware.

As Es and I walk down the food aisles the labels bark at us like puppies in a pet store. Buy Me! Take Me Home! I'm Good for You! I'm Organic! I'm Natural! I'm Nature's Own! I'll Make You Happy! Es disregards the noise and points out the dangers on every shelf and the pedigree of every label.

We all have a mortal fear of cholesterol and the food manufacturers know this. Es picks up a liquid creamer that says in big letters "No Cholesterol." Of course it contains no cholesterol—cholesterol is found only in foods of animal origin, so a "No Cholesterol" label can be put on anything made of vegetables, including products made with artery-clogging saturated fat. This creamer may have no cholesterol but a closer look at the label reveals that it has more fat calories than whole milk.

In aisle six, the home of crackers and snacks, Es picks up a bag of "low-fat" chips that have only twenty calories per serving. Upon closer inspection, the fine print reveals that a "serving" as defined by the manufacturer is three chips. This is not very "low-cal" when you consider that it would take a gross of these microchips to put a dent in your appetite. Es reminds me to check serving size. One size doesn't fit all. What appears to be low in calories often isn't.

As we pass the prepackaged cold cuts in the refrigerator case Es picks up a package of Ball Park franks that scream "97% Fat Free." True. But that figure is based on the percent of fat by weight. It may be 97 percent fat-free but it still can get 80 percent of its calories from fat. Ball Park franks are guaranteed to give you a ball park figure.

In the produce department near the salad greens Es shows me a bottle of "light" olive oil. She points out that "light" means nothing. "Light" olive oil has the same number of calories and fat as butter. They are both fats. A truly light or lean food gets fewer than 30 percent of its calories from fat.

When we arrive at the cheese island a young girl dressed like a milk maid is giving out free samples of "lean" crackers. Es tries one. "This tastes too good to be true." She takes another. It leaves a shiny coating on her fingers. "That's fat" says Es. And that's that.

As we cruise down the aisles we pass packages with big bold letters telling us it's "organic" and "nature's own" and "all natural." This is all nonsense. We are all "organic" and "nature's own." About the only thing that isn't all natural is a henna rinse, a facelift, and a zircon diamond. This stuff should be arrested for impersonating health food. Read the labels. The main ingredient is listed first. If you don't like what you see, move on. Sometimes the product looks perfectly harmless but if you don't look carefully the ingredients can be as deadly as a Japanese blowfish. Before you check out, check out the labels. And after you find either the nonfat or low-fat version of everything you want, leave, which is exactly what Es and I do.

Es was not going to be done in by her diet. Even when we eat out at one of those early bird specials, Es has a game plan. While the other diners are consuming more calories than the national debt, Es remains calm and in control. She will not allow her appetite to overpower her heart. She studies the menu very carefully, completely avoiding the buttered, breaded, creamed, browned, or deep-fried, and she limits her choices to the broiled, grilled, roasted, steamed, poached, or baked entrees. She decides on the grilled chicken breast and then negotiates with Heidi, our waitress, to have it served skinless and with no oil.

Es's new life-style was rubbing off on Irv. When he ordered the fish he had them put the sauce on the side so he could control the portions, and at the salad bar he knew when to say when. We all had dessert because it came with the dinner. Even Es went off her pastry wagon and had a sliver of Key Lime pie. "I'll walk an extra forty minutes tomorrow," she pledged. While we were finishing dinner some of the earlier early birds were waddling out, taking their heart attacks home in a doggie bag. You wonder how many bites they are away from the big one. For how many will this early bird special be the Last Supper?

In the week that I was in Florida I joined Es and her cronies every morning as they tried to walk off the effects of a lifetime's worth of abuse and neglect. They accepted the wrinkles, the bags, the flab, and the whole rotten mess as just a natural part of growing old. They expected to be sick, to spring a leak, to have more aches and pains than discount coupons. It comes with the condo. For these women long past menopause this is a time of self-discovery. They are discovering that maybe menopause, not just old age, had something to do with the softening of their bones and the hardening of their arteries.

These old veterans of menopause spent their middle age in the dark ages of menopause. They lived in a time when doctors chain-smoked, put saccharin in their coffee, asbestos in their siding, and knew almost nothing about nutrition unless you had beri-beri or rickets. These medicine men considered menopause a "woman's problem," not a real medical problem. Women who complained were considered emotional cripples and doctors usually paid very little attention to them. If a woman made a pest of herself she was often kept busy with tons of tranquilizers, truckloads of hormones, or the removal of her uterus, which at the time was the vaginal equivalent of a frontal lobotomy.

The male medical community had no idea of the effect menopause would have on women later in life. But since they weren't getting hot flashes and dry vaginas, they really weren't all that interested in the answer. With this as the prevailing attitude, it was better for a woman to ignore her symptoms than have to deal with a doctor who thought of her as an unstable, estrogen-starved, emotionally handicapped, socially worthless burden on society. Menopausal women were to be pitied. They were a subspecies lower than the homeless. They were the hormoneless. So women like Es ignored their symptoms, hoping they would go away. Unfortunately, menopause affects some three hundred body functions, and the problems that begin with menopause don't go away. There is nothing psychosomatic about heart disease, cancer, and osteoporosis. There is no such thing as mind over menopause. Many of the problems Es and her friends are trying to walk off now could have been prevented then. They didn't have to be casualties of menopause.

Fortunately, we have a greater opportunity to deal physically and emotionally with menopause than did our parents. They didn't have the luxury of climacteric medicine and full-service menopause clinics. We do. Many of the problems of menopause can be prevented if handled early enough. If you are postpuberty, consider yourself premenopausal. Make sure you get plenty of calcium during adolescence along with a healthy diet and exercise. Don't smoke! It's bad for everything. When you are twenty start having annual pelvic exams and Pap smears and do monthly breast self-exams. At thirty-five, estrogen

production begins to decline so get a series of tests annually to determine if you are at risk for heart disease and
get a baseline mammogram and a bone-density test if you
think you are at risk for osteoporosis. If you are overweight do something about it immediately. I am not talking about dark colors and vertical stripes. I am talking
about a low-fat, low-cholesterol diet and aerobic exercise
at least three times a week. The right diet can cut the risk
of cancer by 50 percent, and if you are only 10 percent
over your ideal weight you stand a 30 percent higher
chance of a heart attack. After thirty-five, do weekly
rather than monthly breast self-exams to stay in touch
with your body. Also, get a mammogram every two or
three years until fifty. After fifty, mammograms should be
done every year.

It is never too early to start, and for Es and her
friends it's never too late. Eubie Blake said shortly before
he died at one hundred, "If I'd known I was gonna live
this long, I'd have taken better care of myself." You will
and you should.

ELEVEN

New Beginnings

The phone rings. It is my mother. While visiting my sister she fell and broke her pelvis in two places. "One minute I was walking, the next minute I took a big flop and landed in Emergency. I don't know what hit me." I do. "Mom, what hit you was osteoporosis. Now when you fall things break." She is not listening, she is denying. "It could have happened to anybody. The carpet was loose. If it wasn't your sister's house I would sue them for everything." She tells me that she will be laid up for six to eight weeks, but all she is really concerned about now that she can't get around is who is going to get her her cigarettes. She doesn't get it. I've seen her more upset when she ran into friends when she wasn't wearing makeup. I'm about to tell her once again to stop smoking when she says, "And don't tell me to stop smoking." I tell her anyway. "Mom, if you keep smoking those Camels, soon you're going to look like one. If you don't stop smoking and drinking coffee and start exercising and taking better care of yourself you're not only going to be in bed but also dead." She almost buys it until she realizes that she is my mother. "Don't lecture me, Gayle. You are talking to your mother. You want to be disrespectful, call your father."

Normally, this response would frighten me enough to back off and change the subject to something more benign like oat bran or Richard Simmons. This time I don't. In the past we had avoided the facts of life. Now we had to face them. "Mom, you may not agree, but a broken pelvis and osteoporosis are far more serious than being in an accident without clean underwear. You've got to change your life-style or you may not recover." She already has it figured out. "I'm way ahead of you. I'm already doing something. I'm getting nonskid mats, putting grab bars in the bathroom, and night lights everywhere. No more high heels and walking when it's icy. I'm even going to get one of those 'I fell and can't get up' services that they advertise on TV." I am not impressed. "Mom, get serious. Sensible shoes and avoiding waxy buildup aren't enough. If you don't listen to me you'll never get out of bed. This is not a boil. This is osteoporosis."

The call ended the way they all do, with the usual clichés like "If I didn't love you I wouldn't be saying this" and "Stop thinking about yourself, think about me." Only this time it had real meaning and substance. And importance. It was time for us to both grow up.

When I hang up the phone I realize that I have just had an historical conversation with my mother. For the first time in our lives we have been talking about a subject that affects both of us in a way nothing else has. This is not mother and daughter talking about money, husbands, and shopping. This was two women talking about a common enemy—osteoporosis. I no longer feel like my mother's baby. I am more like her contemporary. The generation gap has closed. When I was five and she was twenty-five we were miles apart. Now, when she is seventy and I am fifty, we are practically neighbors. The only thing that separates us is a hairline fracture. I'm nothing like my mother; now I'm everything like her. If this could happen to her, it could happen to me. I am on her genetic conga line. Heredity is a major factor in osteoporosis. To the best of my knowledge, about the only thing that can't be transmitted genetically is sterility. They say the apple doesn't fall far from the tree, and my mother the tree just fell from osteoporosis.

It has been a year since my last bone-density test. I don't feel any different. But neither did my mother. I remind myself that you're not supposed to; that's not how it works. Osteoporosis can steal your calcium in broad daylight and no alarm goes off. It can be taking it right out of your bones and nobody calls 911. I immediately call and make an appointment for another bone-density test. Same clinic, same technicians, same technologist, same nurse, different results. This time I have lost 7 percent of my bone mass. I am sick. I am reminded that 90,000 osteoporotic women die each year from complications from broken bones, and that osteoporosis begins not in our seventies and eighties but long before.

I am running out of time. I have lost 7 percent of bone this year. Will I lose another 7 percent next year or will it be 14 percent? How long before my bones turn to tapioca and my body has the flexibility of melba toast? How long before I become another little old person peering over the steering wheel of a full-sized car? Parents are the ghosts of Christmas future and from what I've seen my future looks short and porous. My mother's legacy is osteoporosis. I would have preferred jewelry, cash, and a house in the country.

I am well aware of the facts and figures of osteoporosis. The fact is that I can figure on getting osteoporosis if I don't do something soon. In the past year I have tried to take a natural approach to menopause. I was open to everything—noodles, needles, teas, tinctures, touch, massages, mantras, manipulation, meditation, medication, lotions, potions, New Age, Old World, ayurvedic, holistic, even mystic. I consumed packets of pills, pounds of supplements, gallons of oils, bushels of herbs, thousands of dollars, and I still lost 7 percent of bone. I have tried all the alternative approaches and every over-the-counter counter-culture remedy, but I am afraid there is no alternative to estrogen for osteoporosis. No amount of fresh air, healthy food, or meditation will prevent bone loss when the production of estrogen stops. There are no miracles. There is no menopause fairy. There is only estrogen and no amount of exercising, square dancing, and do-si-doing will take its place in preventing osteoporosis. I am not going to second-guess what I have done but I will second-guess what I don't do. That's why I have decided to take estrogen pills—the full course of HRT.

I wouldn't think of taking hormones just for my hot flashes and I definitely wouldn't take them to make my skin moist or my hair thicker. I'm not taking HRT for vanity. I'm taking it for sanity. I know what HRT can do for me and I know what it can do to me. If I don't want to wind up like my mother, I have no choice. I must be realistic. I can't tough out osteoporosis. It will take more than backbone to get bone back. It will take HRT. I don't want to surrender my body to medical science, but I prefer that to surrendering my bones to osteoporosis. I know I've got at least another thirty years and I want to live them vertically.

It is September 1, 1990. Today the Bush administration formally recognizes the three Baltic states as independent nations and I formally declare war on osteoporosis. I begin by taking 0.3 mg Premarin tablets, the smallest dose. The pills work with the speed of a glacier. For the first week nothing happens. The third week I start taking 2.5 mg of Provera. It, too, is the lowest dose you can take. The doctor tells me the Provera may cause bloating and I might get a period, but I prefer this to the risk of uterine cancer from taking Premarin alone. That same week the Premarin pills start to work. Fewer hot flashes and night sweats and no vaginal dryness. At the end of the fourth week, I start noticing the effects of the Provera. I get a slight period and I am bloated and squishy and feel like a walking waterbed. I also have PMS and an incredible craving for sweets. When I order chocolate fudge cake in a Chinese restaurant, I decide to pay another visit to my gynecologist.

My gynecologist says if I take Premarin and Provera every day of the month I won't get a period and won't have PMS symptoms. I want to keep my period. I like being without hormones one week every month and my period shows that I'm cleaning myself out. Besides, I like the idea of buying Tampax again. What I don't like is that I am still getting an occasional hot flash and night sweats. My doctor suggests that I increase my dosage to 0.625 mg of Premarin and 5 mg of Provera. He says it will be better for all my symptoms, especially my bones. Along with the increased dosage I take the liver-strengthening herb milk thistle. Estrogen is broken down in the liver and I'm taking no chances.

The increased dosage eliminates the hot flashes and

night sweats, but now I get major PMS symptoms. My craving for sweets reaches neurotic proportions when I scoop the fruit out of the bottom of every raspberry yogurt container in my refrigerator. It does not end there. In a given day I pay no less than thirty visits to the refrigerator. I open and close it so many times that I burn out the bulb inside. My appetite for food is insatiable. Unfortunately my sexual appetite is still nonexistent. I am sexually anorexic. The HRT has eliminated the pain of sex but it has not stimulated my hunger for sex. I have no desire for desire, no passion for passion, no lust for lust.

The world is struggling to keep its passion in check and mine has checked out. My discomfort grows with every movie I see, every song I hear, every book I read. The world is *Basic Instinct* and Mickey Rourke and ice cubes and bondage and unexpurgated and uncut and I am uninterested. The world is the *Kama Sutra* and I am *Good Housekeeping*. The world is hot and tense and savage and I am Walden Pond. The world spends every single waking moment thinking about "it," and most days the thought of sex never even occurs to me. People around me are throbbing, aching, yearning, and craving, and I am dusting and cleaning and washing and shopping. Sex is on everybody's mind but mine. Why can't I be normal and have thirty orgasms a day like everyone else?

It was time to ask a few discreet, tasteful questions about human sexuality. I call my friend Susan. Before she can even say hello I ask, "Do burning, hot, untamed waves of wild eroticism rip through your throbbing, quivering body every waking moment?" She hangs up. She thinks it's an obscene phone call. When I call back she's reluctant to talk but with a little coaxing and a lot of revealing she lets it rip.

When Susan and her husband sent their youngest son off to college, the two of them let loose sexually. They had the house all to themselves and made love in broad daylight on the kitchen table, in the backyard, and even in the family room with the lights on and their eyes open. They did it everywhere and anywhere but Susan soon lost interest. "It was more exciting with the distractions and interruptions and the lack of privacy. Besides, no matter how many times you do it, it still can't fill the hole left when the kids leave. Kids are a full-time job. Sex isn't even a part-time job." Procreation was no longer recreation. It was now work.

Sue might have lost her sex drive but her husband's was still in high gear. And he didn't believe that abstinence makes the heart grow fonder. She didn't think he would leave her for another woman. "He's sixty-two and too smart for that. He knows that if AIDS doesn't kill him, the property settlement after thirty years of marriage will. But he wants his sex and I have absolutely no interest. Right now I want my ego massaged, not my breasts." Sue thought that her lack of libido was a natural part of aging and we weren't meant to have sex if we couldn't have children. Sue's husband didn't agree and wanted them to go to therapy. Sue was reluctant. "I worry about self-discovery because I don't know what I'll discover." She's thinking of pursuing a life of selfless, sexless community service.

Maybe Sue is on to something. Maybe I should get out of sex and into art and politics. Maybe I should just forget about chasing after my lost libido and pursue more neutral activities. I was a sexual mover, maybe I should become a celibate Shaker and live a quiet life of cabinet-making, church suppers, and prayer meetings. Maybe it's time to find new uses for the missionary position. Maybe it's time to talk to someone else.

Marsha was a life-style freak. She tried everything. She went from open marriage to group marriage to failed marriage. From creative divorce to embittered divorce to single parent to single woman. Marsha's last relationship ended when she ran off with her vibrator. Marsha suggests that I test-drive one. "It never gets sick, snores, yells, sulks, rejects, cheats, gets an attitude, hogs the bathroom, needs its 'space,' is too tired, too busy, or out of town." According to Marsha, it's the safest possible sex as long as you don't take it into the bathtub or shower. Currently, Marsha is living with a super-deluxe multi-function vibrator that does everything but take her to dinner and buy her flowers. I thank her for the advice but I don't believe in reliance on an appliance.

My friend Carol told me that I had ISD—Inhibited Sexual Desire. It's the number-one sexual problem of the nineties. Carol knows about these things. She has a very extensive sex library and has thoroughly read and under-lined every page of the *Kama Sutra, The Joy of Sex,* and *Human Sexual Inadequacy.* She even has a signed first edition of *J, the Sensuous Woman.* Carol and her hus-band have tried everything—touch, Esalen, sex surro-gates, Masters and Johnson. They went to seminars, nude encounter groups, and marriage-enrichment weekends. Unfortunately, she and her husband couldn't do the homework. "It was just too much work for too little satisfaction. To have maybe two good minutes in bed it took us hundreds of hours of therapy and more money than a California divorce. The truth is I get more aroused by a cup of Sanka." When I get off the phone I buy a jar of Sanka. I also try oysters, black olives, and green M&M's. None work. I make an appointment with my doctor to find out what magic potion modern medicine has for my lackluster libido.

My doctor recommends Estratest. It is a combina-tion of estrogen and the male hormone testosterone. Tes-tosterone triggers emotional desire in both men and women. A woman's testosterone level can drop by one-third after menopause or reproductive surgery. I am to take Estratest in place of Premarin. He tells me there might be some side effects like oily skin, and starts me with a full-strength dose.

I go home and wait for the Estratest to kick in. I can't wait to feel the jungle hunger, the untamed passion, the wildly erotic surges of hormones, and the rush of blood to my genitals. I do the mundane daily chores as I await the arrival of the quivering, aching, thunderous passion that will soon be ripping through my throbbing, frenzied, boiling, fiery, steamy, pulsating, palpitating body. After much anticipation and many false starts, I finally get an itch, an urge, a desire. It is working! The earth isn't shaking, mountains aren't moving, but excavation has definitely begun.

In the next few weeks my libido grows tremendously but so does the hair on my upper lip. I now have a five-o'clock shadow. I worry about all these male hormones raging through my body. I like having my libido back but I don't want to have to shave every time we make love. The more Estratest I take, the more energy I get. Too much energy. Male energy. I feel like an animal and I'm starting to look like one. A furry one. This stuff is too powerful. I'm afraid if I continue I'll start drinking beer, watching football all day, spitting, reading the *Playboy Advisor*, and lying about the size of my breasts. I have a good mind to pay a visit to my gynecologist and kick his butt. For the safety of my doctor, my husband, and the entire free world, we reduce the dosage to half strength and it works. Our sex life is now somewhere between *Basic Instinct* and *Honey, I Shrunk the Kids*. It is at a level we can handle comfortably and we both are very satisfied.

* * *

I had been on HRT for about a year and the results were amazing. I no longer had hot flashes, night sweats, PMS, heart palpitations, a dry vagina, and loss of libido. My cholesterol levels were never better, my bone density had increased by four percent, my hair stopped falling out, my skin was moister, I had better muscle tone, I was sleeping, and I had great energy. My doctor was happy with my progress; I was ecstatic. My life had turned around and I was my old self again, or so I thought.

One evening I am driving home alone. I stop for a light, glance around, and notice a couple of teenagers making out like crazy in the car next to me. My windows are rolled up but I can still feel their heat. I try not to notice, to ignore their rubbing, hugging, touching, and groping—but I can't. I am as riveted to them as they are to each other. They are too involved with their own hormones to know that I or anything else in this world exists. When by some miracle of nature and instinct their bodies are notified that the light has changed, they unlock and speed off fused together behind the wheel like some two-headed freak of nature.

After they drive off and the lust has settled, I just sit in my car shocked, startled, and overwhelmed by the heat and intensity inside that other car. This was not a movie or a TV commercial. This was not fiction or a reenactment. This was real life. The experience made me really uncomfortable, very embarrassed, and a little weepy. It was a feeling that I remember very well but had completely forgotten. It reminds me of the good old days before the great chill of menopause.

It reminds me of my first encounter with my hormones. The lights, the bells, the whistles, the itch, the rush, the crush of adolescence. In many ways adolescence and menopause are similar. Adolescence is an awkward age. And menopause is awkward aging. Both are very confusing times, filled with fear, anxiety, guilt, grief, and anger. There are mood swings and attitude shifts. Moments of total security followed by total insecurity. As a teenager I was uncomfortable, insecure, and isolated. I didn't know where I was headed and I feel the same now. It all seems so familiar. It seems like menopause is the adolescence of old age. Yet it isn't at all.

When I was a teenager there were rules and rights and wrongs and dos and don'ts. That has changed. I might not have the libido of my youth but I have more freedom and more wisdom. Now I make my own rules and determine my own destiny.

Youth is wasted on the young. Not menopause. Menopause is for adults only. Kids aren't equipped to handle it. The changes are too cerebral, too advanced, too complicated; the pleasures far too subtle. Menopause is a job for a woman, not a girl. Adolescence is for adolescents. I don't want the chaos and the madness and the self-involvement and dependency of adolescence. I don't want to depend on anybody. I want to be propelled by my brain, not my hormones, by my mind, not my body. I don't want to be my old self, that hot little out-of-control girl who just drove off. I want to be a new woman and I welcome the change. Menopause isn't the end of the road but the beginning of a new adventure.

Some Change-of-Life Savers

FROM CHAPTER FOUR The Hot Tip

Hormone replacement therapy (HRT) refers to the combined use of estrogen and progesterone to treat menopausal symptoms.

BENEFITS OF HRT

- Eliminates hot flashes, night sweats, and insomnia.
- Relieves vaginal dryness and painful sexual intercourse.
- Reduces the risk of cardiovascular disease and stroke.
- Prevents osteoporosis.
- Treats early menopause (before age 40) due to surgery.
- Promotes a sense of well-being and an improved quality of life.
- Increases muscle tone.
- Results in younger-looking skin.

POSSIBLE SIDE EFFECTS OF HRT

- bloating
- cramping
- fluid retention, weight gain
- breast tenderness
- nausea
- depression
- severe mood swings

POSSIBLE CONTRAINDICATIONS

- history of uterine or breast cancer
- high blood pressure
- blood clots in the veins or lungs
- liver disease
- gallstones and gallbladder disease
- diabetes
- stroke
- migraine headaches
- large uterine fibroids
- endometriosis
- varicose veins

HOW HRT IS ADMINISTERED

- oral tablet
- transdermal patch
- vaginal cream

Transdermal Patch—dispenses the required dose of estrogen when applied to the skin twice a week.

ADVANTAGES

- Women with liver disease, high blood pressure, gallbladder disease, or thrombophlebitis may still be able to take estrogen without the negative consequences of stimulating liver proteins.

DISADVANTAGES

- May cause skin irritation in some women.
- May not improve cholesterol levels to the same degree as the oral route because of bypassing the liver, which affects HDL ("good") cholesterol.
- May not adhere properly in humid climates.

Vaginal Cream—applied locally for a few days a week.

ADVANTAGES

- Use of this cream will relieve a dry vagina and improve lubrication for intercourse.

DISADVANTAGES

- Unpredictable rate of absorption into the adrenal circulation.

Dr. Brown's Calcium Content List

	Portion	Calcium Content (mg.)
DAIRY PRODUCTS		
Milk		
Whole	1 cup	288
Low-fat 2%	1 cup	297–313
Skim	1 cup	302–316
Low-fat dry (powdered)	¼ cup	384
Evaporated	½ cup	318
Calcimilk	1 cup	500
Yogurt		
Low-fat plain	1 cup	415
Fruit-flavored low-fat	1 cup	345
Whole-milk	1 cup	275
Cheese		
Swiss	1 oz.	262
Provolone	1 oz.	213
Mozzarella	1 oz.	145
Romano	1 oz.	150
Parmesan	1 oz.	136
Feta	1 oz.	100
Brie	1 oz.	52
Ricotta	4 oz.	256
Cottage, low-fat	1 cup	204
Cottage, regular	1 cup	131

Dr. Brown's Calcium Content List *(continued)*

	Portion	*Calcium Content (mg.)*
FISH AND SEAFOOD		
Clams, steamed or canned	8 oz.	121
Mackerel, canned	8 oz.	552
Lobster	1 lb.	300
Oysters, raw (13–19 medium-size)	8 oz.	226
Salmon, sockeye, canned (with bones)	8 oz.	587
Sardines, canned	3½ oz.	259
Shrimp, canned	3½ oz.	115
Tuna, canned	3 oz.	6
Flounder, baked	4 oz.	28
FRUIT		
Blackberries	1 cup	46
Dates, dried, cut, or pitted	½ cup	52
Figs, dried, cut	5 medium	126
Orange	1 medium	58
Raisins, dried, seedless	½ cup	48
Banana	1 medium	10
Apple, raw	1 large	10
Apricots, dried, uncooked, fresh	1 cup	90
	3 medium	20
Watermelon (4 × 8″)	1 wedge	30

NOTES

Dr. Brown's Calcium Content List *(continued)*

	Portion	*Calcium Content (mg.)*
VEGETABLES		
Arugula	½ cup	309
Bok choy, fresh	1 cup	250
Broccoli, fresh, cooked	1 cup	140
frozen	1 cup	100
Bean sprouts	1 cup	20
Beets, cooked	1 cup	25
Black beans	1 cup	270
Garbanzo beans, canned	1 cup	150
Red kidney beans	1 cup	75
Carrot juice	½ cup	83
Collards, fresh, cooked	1 cup	300
frozen	1 cup	150
Corn, fresh	1 ear	5
Kale, fresh, cooked	1 cup	210
frozen	1 cup	160
Mustard greens, fresh, cooked	1 cup	190
Okra pods, fresh, cooked	10	100
Potato, baked	1 medium	15
french fries	10	10
chips	10	10
Sweet potato, baked, with skin	1 medium	40
Tomato	1 large	25
Turnip greens fresh, cooked	1 cup	250
frozen	1 cup	200

Dr. Brown's Calcium Content List *(continued)*

	Portion	Calcium Content (mg.)
NUTS AND SEEDS		
Almonds, dried	½ cup	170
roasted, salted	½ cup	185
Brazil nuts	½ cup	130
Cashew nuts	½ cup	30
Peanut butter (commercial)	¼ cup	35
Pecans, raw	½ cup	35
Sesame seeds, dry	½ cup	85
Sesame seed, meal	¼ cup	270
Sunflower seeds	½ cup	90
Walnuts, raw	½ cup	60
MEAT AND POULTRY		
Chicken, broiled	3 oz.	7
Duck	3 oz.	9
Pork chop, thick	3 oz.	8
Turkey, roasted	3 oz.	9
Beef, sirloin steak	3 oz.	10
Frankfurter, beef, 7″ long	1	6

NOTES

Dr. Brown's Calcium Content List *(continued)*

MISCELLANEOUS FOODS	Portion	Calcium Content (mg.)
Blackstrap molasses	1 tablespoon	140
Soybean nuts	½ cup	136
Soy sauce	2 tablespoons	89
Corn muffin	1 average	50
Cheeseburger	1 average	152
Tofu	4 oz.	150
Tortillas	2	120
Donuts	1	6–25
Graham crackers	1	6
Gingersnaps	1	5
Beer	1 quart	41

A Bone-Chilling
Experience

Osteoporosis, or porous bone, is a disease characterized
by low bone mass and structural deterioration of bone
tissue, leading to an increased susceptibility to fractures
of the hip, spine, and wrist.

RISK FACTORS* FOR DEVELOPMENT OF OSTEOPOROSIS
INCLUDE THE FOLLOWING:

- being female
- sedentary life-style
- early menopause
- inadequate calcium intake
- smoking
- alcohol consumption
- steroid medications
- history of scoliosis
- Caucasian or Asian
- petite, thin build
- family history of osteoporosis
- postmenopausal

*Risk factors are a condition. You may have many risk factors and still not
develop osteoporosis. The only way to determine if you have osteoporosis is by
taking a bone-density test.

NOTES

CALCIUM REQUIREMENTS
(RECOMMENDED DAILY ALLOWANCES)

Children up to 11 years	800 mg.
Teens and young adults	1200 mg.
Adults, 25 and older	800 mg.
Pregnant and nursing women	1200 mg.
Postmenopausal women	1500 mg.
Women on HRT	1000 mg.

CALCIUM ABSORPTION IS DECREASED OR HINDERED BY
THE FOLLOWING:

- lack of exercise
- frequent use of laxatives and other medicines that cause the intestinal contents to pass rapidly through the body
- excessive phosphorous intake, as from sodas
- a high-protein diet (increases excretion of calcium in the urine and inhibits calcium absorption from the intestines)
- phytic acids, found in many grains
- oxalic acid, found in spinach, beet greens, Swiss chard, and parsley (the oxalic acid in these foods binds only the calcium in that particular food and does not interfere with calcium from a different food that is eaten at the same meal; for example, if you eat a spinach-cheese omelet, the calcium from the spinach will not be absorbed but the calcium from the cheese will be)

- excessive sodium intake—too much salty food robs the body of calcium
- overuse of caffeine—11 mg. of calcium are lost every time you drink a cup of coffee

PREVENTING OSTEOPOROSIS

Building strong bone, especially before the age of 35, may be the best defense against developing osteoporosis, and a healthy life-style is the best preventative:

- Eat a balanced diet rich in calcium
- Exercise regularly, especially weight-bearing activities
- Limit alcohol intake
- Don't smoke
- Ask your physician about hormone replacement therapy if you have had an early or surgically induced menopause
- Have a baseline bone-density test when you reach menopause

SOME BONE-CHILLING FACTS

- Osteoporosis affects one in four women, and one in nine men in the United States
- 1.3 million osteoporosis fractures occur annually
- Approximately 1 to 2 percent of the population over 65 will sustain a hip fracture annually. More than

250,000 hip fractures occur every year because of
osteoporosis. The overall medical costs exceed seven
billion dollars a year

- Between the ages of 25 and 50 Americans lose up to
a third of the total calcium in their skeletons without
being aware of it

- Forty percent of all women will have at least one
spinal fracture by the time they reach 80

- Fifteen percent of white women 50 years and older
will fracture a wrist

- About 15 percent of white women will fracture a hip
at some time during their lives

- Individuals suffering hip fractures have a 5 to 20 percent greater risk of dying within the first year following that injury than others in their age group

- As many as 50,000 people die each year as a result of
hip fractures

- Among those who were living independently prior to
a hip fracture, 15 to 25 percent are still in long term–
care institutions a year after the injury

- Seventy-five percent of all osteoporosis is caused by a
nutritional deficiency

FACTS ABOUT CALCIUM

1 Calcium is a natural tranquilizer and tends to calm
the nerves.
2 Calcium has been successfully used in the treatment
of osteoporosis.

3 Calcium has been beneficial in the treatment of cardiovascular disorders.

4 Calcium, magnesium, and vitamin D have helped overcome problems of menopause, irritability, insomnia, and headaches.

5 Calcium can help prevent premenstrual tension and menstrual cramps.

6 Calcium can help alleviate arthritis and rheumatism.

7 Calcium helps to build and maintain bones and teeth.

8 Calcium is essential for healthy blood.

9 Calcium helps regulate the heartbeat.

10 Calcium assists in the process of blood clotting.

11 Calcium helps prevent too much acid or too much alkali accumulating in the blood.

12 Calcium plays a part in muscle growth, muscle contraction, and nerve transmission.

13 Calcium helps regulate the passage of nutrients in and out of cell walls.

14 We are generally more deficient in calcium than any other mineral.

15 Experiments show that chocolate and cocoa prevent calcium assimilation.

16 Some signs of calcium deficiency in children are: unpleasant dispositions, temper tantrums, and frequent, fretful crying.

17 Adults show calcium deficiencies through nervous habits such as finger tapping and tensing of the foot or swinging the foot when the leg is crossed. They become impatient and snap at their loved ones. They are easily annoyed, jump at slight noises, and often are grouchy. They become restless and cannot sit still for long.

Michael Abhaile's Cordon Bleu Cross Bone-Building Recipes

TERIYAKI TEMPEH STIR-FRY

2 tbsp toasted sesame oil
1 tempeh, thawed, sliced, and marinated in tamari
¼ cup fresh ginger, chopped
4 shiitake mushrooms, sliced
2 tbsp mirin

6 scallions, cut in two-inch pieces
1 tsp brown rice vinegar
½ cup stock
1 tbsp arrowroot

Heat oil in wok or skillet; add tempeh and brown on both sides. Add ginger and mushrooms, sautéing for 2 minutes. Add remaining ingredients and stir-fry one minute more. *Serves 4.*

BETTER BONES AND GARDEN SALAD

1 cup dry medium-grain brown rice
2½ cups pure water, with pinch of sea salt
1 carrot, sliced
¼ head cauliflower, in florets
½ cup arame, soaked
¼ head broccoli, in florets

1 yellow squash, sliced
1 daikon radish, sliced
2 tbsp toasted sesame oil
2 tbsp tamari
2 scallions (garnish)
¼ cup sesame seeds, toasted (garnish)
¼ cup pumpkin seeds, toasted (garnish)

(continued)

Cook rice in salted water and cool. Steam vegetables, first carrot and cauliflower, then softer vegetables. Reserve all water for stock. Whisk tamari into toasted sesame oil slowly until they are creamy. Toss all ingredients together lightly, and garnish with scallions and seeds. *Serves 4.*

HIJIKI YAM BALL BONE-BUILDER

2 large yams
½ cup dry hijiki
2 tbsp fresh ginger, grated
½ cup roasted tahini

1 onion, chopped
2 tbsp tamari
1 cup sesame seeds
2 tsp toasted sesame oil

Bake yams at 350° about 1 hour or until tender. Reserve. Soak hijiki in water for 20 minutes. Blend ginger with tahini. Sauté onion in sesame oil until onion is brown at edges; add tamari. Transfer sautéed onion to tahini blend. Peel and mash (or blend) yams and add to bowl. Add soaked hijiki to bowl. Mix well. Toast sesame seeds in oven. Form yam mixture into small balls and roll in toasted sesame seeds to cover. Serve warm or at room temperature. *Makes 8 balls.*

BONE, SWEET BONE LEMON APRICOT KANTEN

2 cups apple juice
¼ cup raisins
½ cup apricots, sliced
   rind of ½ lemon

pinch of salt
2 tbsp agar-agar flakes
lemon (garnish)

Simmer juice, dried fruits, lemon rind, and salt together for 10 minutes. Remove from heat, add agar-agar, and pour into bowls or mold. Chill. Serve with lemon garnish. *Serves 4.*

Calcium Content of Seaweeds

SEAWEED	Portion	Calcium Content (mg.)
agar-agar	2 oz.	200
arame	2 oz.	575
dulse	3½ oz.	213
hijiki	2 oz.	700
kelp	3½ oz.	942
kombu	2 oz.	400
nori	3½ oz.	188
wakame/alaria	3½ oz.	1100

Kegel Exercises
for Strengthening and Toning
Vaginal Muscles

These exercises should be started in your teens. But it is never too late to learn how to contract and control the pelvic floor muscles. To locate your PC muscles, the next time you go to the bathroom practice starting and stopping the flow of your urine. The muscles that are doing the contracting are the PC muscles. Once you learn the location of these muscles and can control them without urinating, you can do your kegel exercises anytime and anywhere you're in the mood.

To help you to contract your PC muscles correctly, here are some techniques. You don't have to strain for these exercises to work. And remember to keep breathing steadily while doing them.

Let's kegel . . .

THE CLINCH

Contract the PC muscles and hold tightly for 2–3 seconds, then relax. Repeat 10 times, gradually working up to 20 repetitions per day.

THE FLUTTER

Contract and release the PC muscles as rapidly as you can, so that you get a feeling that your muscles are fluttering. Do this 25–30 times a day and work up to 200 per day.

THE ELEVATOR

While sitting or lying on your back, take a deep breath and pretend you are riding an elevator. Starting at the bottom floor with an anal contraction, move up along the PC muscles until you reach the vaginal area, tightening up the muscles until you reach the top floor. Then gradually relax the muscles, "floor by floor," until you return to the bottom floor. Repeat this trip 6 times, 3 times a day.

THE FAUCET

To check muscle tone and strength, while sitting or lying on your back push down as if ejecting something from your vagina. Then, tighten the PC muscles. A word of caution: For obvious reasons, do not attempt this exercise in a public place with a full bladder.

Happy kegeling!

FROM CHAPTER TEN The Heart of the Matter

1 More than 500,000 American women die of cardio-vascular disease each year.
2 Women get as many heart attacks as men.
3 By age fifty-five heart disease is women's #1 killer.
4 Estrogen boosts the level of HDL ("good" cho-lesterol). After menopause, when estrogen levels decline, its protection is lost and the risk of heart attack increases dramatically in women.
5 When women do have heart attacks, they are twice as likely as men to die within the first few weeks.
6 Nearly one-third of all heart attacks in women go undiagnosed.
7 Thirty-nine percent of women who have a heart attack will die within a year. If they survive the first year, they are twice as likely to have a second attack.
8 By walking 30 minutes every day, you could reduce your risk of dying from heart disease by 50 percent.
9 The right diet can cut your risk of cancer by 50 percent.

224

10 If you are 10 percent over your ideal weight, you stand a 30 percent higher chance of having a heart attack.

REDUCING YOUR RISK OF HEART ATTACK

- The desirable cholesterol level for healthy adults is 200 or less.
- LDL ("bad" cholesterol) should be below 130.
- HDL ("good" cholesterol) should be between 50–60.
- Dietary fat intake should be less than 30 percent of your daily calories.
- No more than 10 percent of your daily calories should come from saturated fats.
- Limit your cholesterol intake to below 300 mg. a day.
- For every 1 percent cut you make in cholesterol, there is a 2 percent drop in heart attack risk.

PREVENTION: WHAT YOU CAN DO FOR YOURSELF

- During adolescence, get plenty of calcium, adhere to a healthy diet, exercise, and don't smoke.
- In your 20's, start getting annual pelvic exams, Pap smears, and monthly breast exams.
- At thirty-five—when estrogen production begins to decline—get tested annually to determine if you're

at risk for heart disease and get a baseline
mammogram and a bone-density test if you think
you're at risk for osteoporosis.

- At thirty-five, do a weekly rather than a monthly
breast self-exam.
- Get a mammogram every 2 to 3 years until age
fifty.
- After fifty, mammograms should be done every
year.
- Eat a low-fat, low-cholesterol diet and do aerobic
exercises at least 3 times a week.

ES'S TOP **10** WAYS TO CUT FAT AND AVOID
INTENSIVE CARE:

1 Avoid completely tropical oils (saturated fats) such
as cocoa, butter, coconut oil, palm oil, and palm
kernel oils.
2 Go easy on the good oils (monosaturated fats),
such as olive oil and canola oil. They may be good
for your heart, but they are bad for your waistline.
They have the same fat calories as the bad oil.
There are 120 fat calories in just 1 tablespoon of oil
no matter whether it's saturated or unsaturated.
Just 4 tablespoons of any oil should be your daily
limit for fats.
3 Stay away from processed meats—sausage,
bologna, salami, and hot dogs. Seventy to eighty

percent of their total calories comes from fat. Even a "low-fat" sausage still gets 60 percent of its calories from fat.

4 Limit yourself to one 3½-ounce portion of lean meat (fish, chicken, etc.) per day. That portion is roughly the size of a deck of cards. Trim away fat. Just by removing the skin from a chicken breast, you can cut the fat calories in half. Stay away from "choice" and "prime" cuts. Choose "select"; it has less fat. Avoid duck and goose and pre-basted turkeys.

5 Go easy on cheeses, which are often fattier than meat. Go easy on eggs also. One large egg yolk contains almost the entire daily allowance for cholesterol (250–275 mg.). An egg white contains no cholesterol and is a good source of protein.

6 Choose low-fat or no-fat dairy products. If you drink 2 glasses of whole milk every day for a year, it will give you about 12 pounds of dietary fat. But 2 glasses of skim milk every day for a year will provide less than a tenth of a pound of fat.

7 Stay away from mayonnaise. It is 99 percent fat, with a little egg yolk—which is 99 percent cholesterol. Eat foods that reduce your cholesterol level: salmon, sardines, tuna, green vegetables, and soybean oil.

8 Do not fry anything. A baked potato is 200 calories;

french-fry it and it is 300. Invest in nonstick cookware and use an aerosol cooking spray.

9 Go easy on salt. The American Heart Association recommends no more than 3000 mg. a day (1 teaspoon has 2,132 mg.). Rinse anything canned under water; it will remove most of the salt. Eat plenty of potassium. It helps remove the salt from your system.

10 Learn how to read food labels.

Index

INDEX

Salt, 182, 215, 228
Scoliosis, 213
Seaweed, 123, 125, 221
Self-image, 154–57
Sex life: and estrogen/HRT, 53, 171,
    196–202, 205; husbands' reactions to
    lack of, 164–68; as a marital prob-
    lem, 18, 151–71; and self-image,
    154–57; substitutes for, 152–53, 198;
    and vaginal dryness, 18, 37, 70,
    110–11, 170–71. *See also* Libido
Skin, 53, 201, 205, 207, 213
Sleep, 38, 108, 133, 140, 201. *See also*
    Insomnia
Smoking: and heart disease, 225; and
    osteoporosis, 66–67, 72, 74–75,
    190–91, 213, 215; and prevention of
    menopausal problems, 188
Steroid medications, 213
Stress. *See* Hypertension
Strokes, 119, 120, 206
Support groups, xvii, 32–36
Syncro Energizer, 116–17

Teeth, 94–95
Teriyaki Tempeh Stir-Fry (recipe), 219
Testosterone. *See* Estratest
Thrombophlebitis, 207

Uterine cancer: bleeding as sign of, 53;
    and estrogen/HRT, 52, 57, 58, 59,
    61, 195, 206; and progesterone, 171
Uterine fibroids, 53, 98, 206

Vagina: examination of, 20–21, 50–51,
    188; itching of, 161; kegel exercises
    for, 160–61, 222–23
Vaginal cancer, 59
Vaginal dryness: and acupuncture, 142;
    and ayurveda, 137; and estrogen/
    HRT, 21, 51, 54, 171, 195, 201, 205,
    207; and herbs, 110–11; natural
    lubricants for, 161; and Replens, 56,
    70; and sex life, 18, 37, 70, 110–11,
    170–71; and vitamin E, 117
Varicose veins, 206
Vegetarianism, 72, 75–76
Visualization, 43–44
Vitamin C, 7, 117
Vitamin D, 83, 217
Vitamin E, 37, 55–56, 70, 117
Vitamins/minerals: and bone-density
    tests, 147, 149; dosages of, 147–48;
    and headaches, 217; and insomnia,
    217; and irritability, 217; and mood
    swings, 117; side effects of, 149; and
    the holistic approach, 145–49. *See
    also specific vitamin or mineral*

Weight problems. *See* Obesity

Yeast infections, 51, 110
Yoga, 111–15, 118–19, 121, 127,
    128–29